Principles
of Social Work Practice
A Generic Practice Approach

HAWORTH Social Work Practice
Carlton E. Munson, DSW, Senior Editor

New, Recent, and Forthcoming Titles:

Gerontological Social Work Supervision by Ann Burack-Weiss and Frances Coyle Brennan

Group Work: Skills and Strategies for Effective Interventions by Sondra Brandler and Camille P. Roman

If a Partner Has AIDS: Guide to Clinical Intervention for Relationships in Crisis by R. Dennis Shelby

Social Work Practice: A Systems Approach by Benyamin Chetkow-Yanoov

Elements of the Helping Process: A Guide for Clinicians by Raymond Fox

Clinical Social Work Supervision, Second Edition by Carlton E. Munson

Intervention Research: Design and Development for the Human Services edited by Jack Rothman and Edwin J. Thomas

Forensic Social Work: Legal Aspects of Professional Practice by Robert L. Barker and Douglas M. Branson

Now Dare Everything: Tales of HIV-Related Psychotherapy by Steven F. Dansky

The Black Elderly: Satisfaction and Quality of Later Life by Marguerite M. Coke and James A. Twaite

Building on Women's Strengths: A Social Work Agenda for the Twenty-First Century by Liane V. Davis

Family Beyond Family: The Surrogate Parent in Schools and Other Community Agencies by Sanford Weinstein

The Cross-Cultural Practice of Clinical Case Management in Mental Health edited by Peter Manoleas

Environmental Practice in the Human Services: Integration of Micro and Macro Roles, Skills, and Contexts by Bernard Neugeboren

Basic Social Policy and Planning: Strategies and Practice Methods by Hobart A. Burch

Fundamentals of Cognitive-Behavior Therapy: From Both Sides of the Desk by Bill Borcherdt

Social Work Intervention in an Economic Crisis: The River Communities Project by Martha Baum and Pamela Twiss

The Relational Systems Model for Family Therapy: Living in the Four Realities by Donald R. Bardill

Feminist Theories and Social Work: Approaches and Applications by Christine Flynn Saulnier

Social Work Approaches to Conflict Resolution: Making Fighting Obsolete by Benyamin Chetkow-Yanoov

Principles of Social Work Practice: A Generic Practice Approach by Molly R. Hancock

Nobody's Children: Orphans of the HIV Epidemic by Steven F. Dansky

Social Work in Health Settings: Practice in Context, Second Edition by Toba Schwaber Kerson and Associates

Principles
of Social Work Practice
A Generic Practice Approach

Molly R. Hancock, MSW

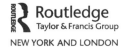

Routledge
Taylor & Francis Group

NEW YORK AND LONDON

First Published by

The Haworth Press, Inc., 10 Alice Street, Binghamton, NY 13904-1580

Published by Routledge
711 Third Avenue, New York, NY 10017
2 Park Square, Milton Park, Abingdon, Oxon, OX14 4RN

Cover design by Marylouise E. Doyle.

Library of Congress Cataloging-in-Publication Data

Hancock, Molly R.
   Principles of social work practice : a generic practice approach / Molly R. Hancock.
      p.   cm.
   Includes bibliographical references and index.
   ISBN 0-7890-0188-8 ISBN: 0-7890-6024-8
   1. Social service. 2. Social service–North America. 3. Social workers–Professional ethics.
I. Title.
HV40.H282   1997
361.3′2–dc20
                                                                                    96-28126
                                                                                        CIP

Publisher's Note
The publisher has gone to great lengths to ensure the quality of this reprint
but points out that some imperfections in the original may be apparent.

This book is dedicated
with my sincere gratitude

to

John F. Boys, MSW (1920-1996)
and
Arthur L. Lesser, MD, FRCP(C), FAPA

At two critical points in my life, they each showed me what
a helping relationship is, giving me a firm place to stand,
while they taught me to know that it was not only safe, but
good, to discover and become more of who I am.

ABOUT THE AUTHOR

Molly R. Hancock, MSW, CSW, is a recently retired counselor for women in Sudbury, Ontario. She was also Associate Professor in the School of Social Work at Laurentian University in Sudbury for several years. Ms. Hancock specializes in working with adult children of dysfunctional families with histories of alcohol, sexual, physical, and psychological abuse. She has also worked extensively with troubled lesbian women as individuals and as couples. She is a member of the Ontario Association of Social Workers and has been active in Association matters locally and provincially for nearly thirty years. Also a member of the Ontario College of Certified Social Workers, the Ontario Social Development Council, and the Canadian Council on Social Development, Ms. Hancock was recently awarded an honorary life membership in the Canadian Association of Schools of Social Work for her distinguished contributions to social work education in Canada.

CONTENTS

Preface

Several generations of social workers–my own included–cut their professional teeth on F. P. Biestek's seminal presentation of professional principles, *The Casework Relationship,* published in 1957. As the title indicates, the work focused specifically on social work with individuals (then called casework), making no mention of group work or community practice. The incorporation of systems theory into social work's theory base in the early 1960s brought about many changes in practice thinking and methods, and this led to a generic practice approach in the teaching curriculum.

With sincere respect for the late Father Biestek's work, my objective in offering this book has been fourfold. First, I wished to preserve some of his timeless insights and sensitive expression. Second, I wanted to demonstrate that the principles he identified were valid and useful in work with client systems of any size. Third, I wished to incorporate some principles that have become intrinsic to practice since Biestek wrote. Lastly, I have attempted to present this material in a configuration that will be readily useable with today's multicultural, multifaith student population.

I am profoundly grateful to Father Biestek, who was still alive when this project was first undertaken, and who gave me not only his approval and permission, but his encouragement.

All the case examples are imaginary, except where I have explicitly cited my own practice. Naturally, most include details from my own or others' experience, but none as presented here replicates any actual case. Distinguishing characteristics of cases from my own practice have been altered where necessary to avoid identification.

Acknowledgments

Many people have given generously of their time, energy, and expertise to help me with this book. First among them is my friend and former colleague at Laurentian University School of Social Work, Dr. Ken Calmain, whose keen mind, unwavering honesty, and editorial eagle eye were invaluable as he painstakingly reviewed and made constructive suggestions for each chapter–sometimes more than once–in draft form. My friend Harry Street, MSW, also contributed valuable editorial suggestions and help at an early stage.

Dr. Joan Newman Kuyek and Laurie McGauley, BA, both gifted and experienced community development workers, contributed immeasurably in consultations about community practice. Leigh McEwen, MSW, gave me of her time and sensitive insight in consultation, as well as invaluable reference material on Palliative Care. Dr. Jennifer Keck of Laurentian University School of Social Work also provided encouragement, helpful suggestions, and some very useful reference material.

Professor Ashley Thomson of Laurentian University Library was always encouraging and helpful in too many ways to list here. Professor Bob Wilson and Dr. Eileen Goltz of the L. U. Library Reference Department and–I think at one time or another almost all–their staff members were a very present help in time of trouble. Unfailingly interested and encouraging, patient and good-humored, at times rescuing me from near despair, they helped me locate many resources, publication dates, and places–the kind of details that are *not* "small" in a project like this, and whose obscurity can sometimes effectively and maddeningly hold up one's progress.

I am very grateful indeed to Loyola University Press for permission to quote extensively from the late Father F. P. Biestek's landmark work on principles of social work practice, *The Casework Relationship,* first published by them in 1957.

Introduction

North American society licenses selected professions, either through legal mandate or institutional sanction, to perform certain functions in defined areas of social need. It is generally accepted that any profession so licensed carries responsibilities that demand, along with technical competence, a value base, usually expressed in a code of ethics. Such a code is considered binding upon those who claim the right to practice the profession.

A study such as the present one, which aims to identify and discuss significant principles of social work practice, must look first at the nature of professional social work. Next, it is important to examine the essence of its value base and code of ethics, and from there to move to the place of such principles as an integral element of practice.

An early definition by The National Association of Social Worker's Commission on Social Work Practice is a useful starting point. They defined social work practice as "a constellation of values, purpose, sanction, knowledge and method" (1958:5). This definition identifies in broad terms the essential components of social work as it is practiced in North America today. We are legitimated by the community's sanction of our activities in certain defined areas of social need. We must carry out our function with a sense and understanding of purpose, basing it upon a body of knowledge, and employing skill in the application of that knowledge in appropriate method; the whole is undergirded by a system of values, consistent with the responsibility entrusted to us.

THE VALUE BASE

Weick states that social work derives its value base in general from a humanistic, democratic, sociopolitical philosophy, while the knowledge base is drawn from the methods of the natural sciences:

1

the latter emphasizing knowledge to be gained from observation and measurement of quantifiable phenomena. (1987:218)

However, Weick warns against the danger she sees of overemphasizing the significance of knowledge vis-à-vis values (1987: 219). Thus in this author's view, while values and knowledge can be separated conceptually, in practice the value base needs to be a strong presence and must at all times influence the application of knowledge in the methods we employ (1983:467). Levy rephrases this notion even more decisively when he states that "formulations of ethical responsibility also constitute a valid form of knowledge" (1972:101).

The same point is expressed somewhat differently by Vigilante, who asserts that:

> ... professional values in social work are more than merely the philosophical base of practice. In proper practice, values are part of the instrumentality of providing service. . . . Professional values permeate decision-making. (1974:40)

Our earliest beginnings–in the Settlement House movement, for example–were rooted in a sense of the universal human need for communal connectedness, a belief that the individual and society were interdependent. Our founders felt that this interdependence laid upon society a certain responsibility to ensure to all its members basic levels of social, economic, and personal health and well-being (Weick, 1987:220).

In the introduction to their anthology of readings on *Fundamentals of Social Work Practice,* Sanders, Kurren, and Fisher identify the professional social workers' obligation to attend to this interdependence in their everyday practice. While their statement summarizes the philosophy that moved our predecessors in the Settlement House movement, they point out its appropriateness in today's practice of social work, stating that:

> ... social work can be viewed as a profession concerned with enhancing the social functioning of individuals in society, of improving social relationships and of *changing social institutions and policies with a view to contributing to the fullest*

possible development of all individuals. (Sanders, Kurren, and Fisher, 1982:2, emphasis added)

It is important that in our eagerness to adopt and apply new learning about the individual struggles of troubled people, we do not lose sight of the fact that for some the origins of their pain may lie in the very nature of a society that systemically obstructs opportunities for some of its members' growth and full participation in the community (Weick, 1987:6). The statement of Sanders, Kurren, and Fisher above points out our professional responsibility of working for social change toward realizing these goals. The problem of fulfilling this responsibility is touched on below.

The increasing development of the profession's psychosocial knowledge had a significant effect on our values. Weick suggests that our philosophy, and in consequence our values, were influenced by changes over time in our "understandings about human beings, society and professional helping" (1987:220). She lists these as follows:

- people have inherent capacity to develop in more fully human ways;
- this development occurs within complex, interactive social and physical environments; and
- professional relationship is one medium through which positive change in both individual and social spheres can occur. (1987:220)

These are fundamental, basic assumptions that form, in part, the foundation of professional practice as it has developed in the second half of this century. Weick's three statements are significant for the examination of values in the context of practice.

VALUES IN PRACTICE

First, all three clearly assume as their baseline the vital interconnectedness of individual and society. The healthy development of the human being is seen to depend upon his or her opportunities to interact with others in the kind of society that would be what I call a healthy place in which to grow people. As mentioned above, many of the values and attitudes of North American society are inimical to such development opportunities for all its members. These values are often expressed in policies and procedures that are demonstrably conducive only to the healthy growth and development of those—predominantly the financially secure—who have the resources, either personal or material or both, with which to establish beneficial linkages in their community. Those who lack such resources are frequently blocked by exclusion[1]–implicit or explicit–from the mainstream of society and thus from opportunities for health-promoting interaction (Weick, 1987:221). It is here that social workers often find themselves in conflict between their primary concern for their clients' well-being and development–an ethical obligation, as will be listed later–and the demands or restrictions of public attitudes or social policy.

Second, in Weick's third "understanding" the professional worker-client relationship is introduced as a significant factor in bringing about change. Biestek, whose seminal work on principles was structured on the centrality of the professional helping relationship, called it "the soul of social casework" (1957:18). In the current generic approach to practice his phrase stands as valid–and as valuable–as when he first wrote it.

Third, implicit in the first statement is the long-held, fundamental professional conviction that human beings have the capacity to change; to change their ways of thinking, feeling, and acting for the achievement of more satisfying personal and social outcomes. In Weick's third statement this concept of change is identified as an essential purpose in social work. This focus upon the process of change is elaborated by Pumphrey when she says:

> Change in a positive direction, for individuals, groups or orga-
> nized societies, may be speeded by active and purposive assis-
> tance or encouragement from others. Change in a negative direc-
> tion may be slowed or prevented by the intervention of others. In
> other words, "helping" is a process of demonstrated validity and
> is a value to be respected in its own right. (1959:43-44)

Here the relationship is again identified as the primary instrument of purposive intervention for achieving positive change. The concept of helping as a value is important in that it validates both our commitment to the helping interventive approach and our professional conviction about the worth of what we do.

The cardinal value that has been given primacy in all the literature on this subject is cited by Siporin as "respect for the worth and dignity of the individual" (1975:75). He further quotes an earlier writer who stated that "It is ultimately in this, in the dignity and worth of man that the philosophy of social work rests" (Younghusband, 1964:106). This all-pervasive concept of individual worth and dignity must characterize the quality of our practice in each and every helping situation, from its inception through its termination.

Biestek stated that this dignity is inherent in the individual and that it cannot in any measure be added to or diminished by any action, achievement or quality of the person (1957:73-74). In light of the many kinds of people in trouble with whom we work, this is a vitally important tenet for social workers. We have been socialized to think of "respect" in terms of its needing to be earned through the display of admirable qualities or superior achievements. But by whatever path of religious faith or philosophical conviction we reach it, we need to believe that every individual is entitled to our respect, because of his or her uniqueness. Their personal characteristics, attributes, or actions should have no bearing on our respect for their unique individuality. The implications for this in practice will be dealt with in detail later; here it is only necessary to state that it needs to be the essential foundation of all decisions about interventive method, whether their impact in the helping process is large or small. It is furthermore the basis of our professional ethics.

SOCIAL WORK ETHICS IN PRACTICE

As noted above, a code of ethics is an essential characteristic of any profession. For social workers, it is that set of statements made by our respective professional bodies (national, state, and provincial associations), that set forth the behavioral obligations laid upon us by the character of the work for which we are mandated by society and to which we are professionally committed. Our ethics must be the ruling guidelines of our behavior in every instance where we act in our professional capacity. But there is nothing absolute or abstract about the profession's ethics; they are shaped by what we are required to do. Levy makes this clear in stating that:

> It is not good conduct in universal terms that makes for ethical conduct in professional practice, it is behavior that is consonant with the requisites of the professional service situation. (1972:96)

Biestek (1957) also affirms this when he writes of the seven practice principles he identifies as springing from the basic human needs of the troubled person, as he or she presents at the point of seeking help or needing service. Thus a study of the essential principles of professional social work must by definition take place within the framework of the professional service situation. When we accept as indispensable the integration of ethics with practice—of values and method—it is patently impossible to separate the practice principles into categories of "ethical" and "technical." Siporin states that

> the distinctions between technical and ethical practice principles are not hard and sharp, because the technical principles are informed by moral considerations and have moral aspects. . . . [The social worker needs] to be both technically competent and morally committed, *to be both efficient and humane.* (1975:114, 116, emphasis added)

From this brief examination of the place of values in the ethical and knowledge framework of the profession, it is useful now to examine how these essential components are translated into practice, how they shape the process of helping, and how they are expressed in the implementation of the principles that are the subject of this study.

THE HELPING PROCESS

Using NASW's earlier statement as a foundation, it is helpful to look at definitions of social work that are more specific in identifying what social work involves and what social workers do. At the practice level, then, Bartlett's definition is valuable in that she identifies the concept of planned and purposeful change as central to practice:

> Social work focuses upon social functioning, i.e., the relation between the coping activity of people and the demands from their environment, . . . [upon] what goes on between people and their environment through the exchange between them, . . . Thus person and situation, people and environment are encompassed in a single concept, which requires that they be constantly reviewed together. Thus the change that social workers effect is *planned with the goal of restoring, maintaining and enhancing the interaction between the person and the environment for the mutual benefit of both.* (1970:104, emphasis added)

Second, her approach of always viewing the person and situation as a single identity incorporates the core of the systems view of human phenomena, which is a cornerstone of today's professional theory. We need to realize that in this view "environment" can be immediate, as in a whole family context, and also distant, to varying degrees, which may include the workplace and the client system's membership and status within the local and the wider community.

Taking this concept of planned change as basic, and drawing on these and other writers' definitions (Siporin, 1975), I believe that in somewhat more specific terms the process of helping in social work practice may be defined as:

> A process that has the goal of bringing about planned change in human situations; the process being a shared endeavor, within a relationship between one or more persons who desire or are under some external pressure to change, and another person or persons designated by professional training and position as having responsibility as agent(s) of change.

In thus describing basic practice, this definition echoes Weick, Biestek, and others in indicating that the relationship between worker and client system is integral to the activity. The description of the activity as being shared identifies further a principle of method, i.e., the active involvement of the client in the process of change. This has become a cardinal principle, as Weick points out, in the profession's evolution as it struggled to free itself from what she terms the "Disease Model." That model embodied the subordination of the "patient" to the professional's diagnosis and the requirement of his or her unquestioning "obedience" in carrying out the prescribed curative measures (1983:468).

It will be noted that both these definitions encompass Bartlett's (1970) concept of a common base of social work practice. In this connection–I have not been able to verify the author–someone wrote that:

> Talk about casework, group work and community work is significant only in describing the number of persons with whom the social worker works and the structure of their inter-relationship. *It is not a significant distinction in terms of what the social worker does.* (emphasis added)

It is from this assumption of a common base of practice with individuals, families, groups, communities, and organizations that the present study of what I believe are basic, essential principles of practice has been undertaken, using Biestek's seminal work as the primary source.

PRINCIPLES OF PRACTICE

I find it practical to group the principles into three categories. First, those that are clearly ethical, in that any breach of these in practice would be seen–and treated professionally–as a breach of the code of ethics, rather than as a failure of competence.

These are:

- respect for the worth and dignity of every human being;
- the worker's primary responsibility is to the client's well-being, not the worker's interests; and
- confidentiality, without which there can be no effective helping relationship.

Second, there is a group of principles that address required qualities to be learned and cultivated by the professional person in the conscious, disciplined use of self–viewing the self as the worker's primary tool in practice:

- responsibility for self-awareness
- controlled emotional involvement
- acceptance
- the nonjudgmental attitude

Third, those which are more clearly principles of method:

- individualization
- the active involvement of the client in the helping process
- purposeful expression of feelings
- client self-determination
- empowerment

In the chapters that follow, each principle will be discussed in the practice context of the helping process, demonstrating the application of each with client systems of varied numerical size. First, a general overview will be offered, paying attention to the application of the principles in the first encounter between worker and clients.

NOTE

1. The term "exclusion" in this context will be seen by some to be inadequate, in light of the perceived harsh reality of policies that–in their view–systemically structure the acceptance of certain levels of poverty and unemployment in society to maintain and enhance the economic status quo. There are those who feel the profession has been politically inept in its approach to social justice issues and consequently ineffective in fulfilling our responsibility for social change. However, it is beyond the scope and purpose of this book to elaborate on this.

REFERENCES

Bartlett, Harriet. (1970). *The Common Base of Social Work Practice*. New York: National Association of Social Workers.

Biestek, Felix P. (1957). *The Casework Relationship*. Chicago, IL: Loyola University Press.

Levy, Charles S. (1972). "The Context of Social Work Ethics." *Social Work,* 17(2):95-101.

National Association of Social Workers. Commission on Social Work Practice. (1958). "Working Definition of Social Work Practice." *Social Work,* 3(2):5-8.

Pumphrey, Muriel W. (1959) *The Teaching of Values and Ethics in Social Work Education.* Vol. 13, A Project Report of the Curriculum Study. New York: Council on Social Work Education. Cited in Sanders, Kurren, and Fisher, 1982.

Sanders, Daniel S., Oscar Kurren, and Joel Fisher. (1982). *Fundamentals of Social Work Practice: A Book of Readings.* Belmont, CA: Wadsworth Publishing Co.

Siporin, Max. (1975). *Introduction to Social Work Practice.* New York: Macmillan

Vigilante, Joseph L. (1974). "Between Values and Science: Education for the Profession During a Moral Crisis, or Is Proof Truth?" *Journal of Education for Social Work,* 10:107-115. Cited in Sanders, Kurrea, and Fisher (1982).

Weick, Ann. (1987). "Re-conceptualizing the Philosophical Perspective of Social Work." *Social Service Review,* 61(2): June, 218-221.

———— (1983). "Issues in Overturning a Medical Model of Social Work Practice." *Social Work,* 28(6):467-471.

Younghusband, Eileen. (1964). *Social Work and Social Change.* London: George Allen and Unwin. Cited in Siporin, 1975:75.

PART I:
THE PRINCIPLES
AND THE SOCIAL WORK ENCOUNTER

Chapter 1

The Ingredients
of Professional Helping

The encounter between social worker and person(s) requesting or referred for help involves, from the very outset, a complex set of attitudes and feelings that each brings to the situation (Biestek, 1957:13-14.) At the point of first contact, we shall be helpful precisely to the degree that we recognize both our own attitudes toward and feelings about this request or need for help and some of the attitudes and feelings these persons may have in this situation. We shall need to understand that the attitudes and feelings that we all bring into the situation are part of the situation's reality and that—from both sides—these may either be constructive or constitute blocks to the beginning of the helping relationship. This situation can involve many variations in these attitudes and feelings; the primary difference is whether the person(s) come voluntarily, or are referred by some other agency.

The situation of the clients' personal need is first manifest within this complex of attitudes and emotions at the point of first encounter. This need immediately demands that we use our practice principles appropriately, as they apply, in the helping situation (Biestek, 1957:14).

THE NEED FOR SELF-AWARENESS

The need for recognition of our own feelings at the point of first contact brings in the principle of responsibility for self-awareness.

For example, how do I feel about a woman who punished her six-year-old son for eating the last of the family's doughnuts by holding the flat of his hand on a heated stove ? If I am human I am angry. How could she do that? It is, however, my professional responsibility to recognize that while my anger is real and valid in the immediate moment, if I am to help this woman I must not let it get in our way. The principle will be discussed in detail later, but for now this example indicates an important principle that is called into play by the need of the client for an objective hearing as we begin the work of bringing about change.

CLIENTS' ATTITUDES AND FEELINGS

The first and most important emotion almost invariably experienced by the client(s) is damaged self-esteem. Their very presence in our office is a painful admission that they have not been able to resolve the problem on their own.

North American culture has traditionally made it very difficult to acknowledge a need for outside help with personal problems. The received wisdom of our culture has indoctrinated us into thinking that if we are really worthwhile people we are able to solve personal problems through our own efforts. This has probably been most difficult for men in our culture, but only somewhat less so for women. This doctrine—I think the word is appropriate—is to some extent being modified at present. There is a beginning acceptance that some life struggles do legitimately require, and respond to, professional intervention. Acceptance or rejection of this trend can vary cross-culturally, but many people still experience to varying degrees the feeling that needing outside help with a personal difficulty is an indication of a "defect of character."

Damaged self-esteem—the feeling of failure, of being a not-okay person for needing to seek our help—is the first emotion shared by almost all our clients as they first come to us. Low self-esteem is present whether the client, individual, family, or organization has sought help voluntarily, or has been referred by a court order (e.g. child protection or criminal process), or has been urged—perhaps pressured—by a parent, pastor, or close friend. In these latter instances the identification and exposure of their problem by others, especially by authority figures, will compound the low self-esteem factor. It can often carry particular meanings, triggering old feelings of inadequacy in not meeting the high expectations of parents, for example. Alternatively, their present situation may serve to confirm a rejecting parent's bitter prophecy: "You'll never amount to anything."

Although there may be some common inner responses to this perception of "failure," each person, group, or organization will perceive their situation in terms that are unique to them. This may reflect the relatively strong or weak influence of family, ethnic, religious group, or community attitudes on this person's or group's perception of themselves as "having failed."

THE AUTHORITY COMPONENT

We need to recognize–and must not ignore–that there is an authority and power component, of varying degree, in all areas of social work (Studt, 1959; Hancock, 1986; Hugman, 1991). Once we have explained clearly to a family coming for therapy the rationale for whole-family sessions, they will perceive that it is our authority of expertise that requires this as the condition of giving the service. This authority is often backed up by the power to refuse service if the family do not meet this condition. The patient in a hospital sees us as having information about community services that makes us "experts" in the area of discharge and homecare, and that we have the power to help them hook into those services. Offenders and neglectful parents are well aware that we have decision-making power, based in legal authority, that can immediately affect their lives and relationships; the adoptive applicants know that our expertise and our position give us the authority to accept or refuse their application for a child; the applicant for social assistance knows that our position gives us the power to approve or reject their claim of eligibility, and thus to affect their security.[1]

The discomfort we may initially feel in accepting the authority and power components in all areas of practice can be alleviated as we first come to accept them as part of the total reality of the helping situation, for the client and for ourselves. Second, we can begin to see these as very often being constructive tools in the helping process, often a means of helping people find what they need to rebuild their lives (Hancock, 1986:128). It is our own attitude toward authority that will make the difference. We need to learn that, constructively used–as a tool and not a weapon–it can be an expression of what I call "responsible caring." Our responsibility for self-awareness will be of critical importance here.

Just as we bring our own feelings about and attitudes toward authority to this aspect of our helping role, so will our clients bring feelings and attitudes stemming from previous experiences with authority figures. Depending upon the nature of these previous experiences, some clients may perceive the authority as overriding the helping component. We shall need to respond sensitively to this as we begin with them.

THE REFERRAL SOURCE

Persons in need of help may come to us in a wide range of different circumstances. The most obvious and first difference, as noted above, is between those who seek help voluntarily and those who come under some external pressure and not of their own volition.

> The Lennard family have come to your agency voluntarily, identifying eight-year-old Kevin's behavior problems at home and in school as "the problem." Kevin is the middle child of three siblings, the first son of the family. Although initially they saw no reason for anyone but Kevin to be involved, with the help of your explanation of its value, they have agreed to come as a family for therapy. Their voluntary request for help does not preclude the loss of self-esteem these parents experience.

Blaming the parents for their children's behavior difficulties– whether at home, at school, or with the law–is virtually an automatic response in our society at the present time. Ours is a society that fundamentally assumes that biological capacity for parenthood automatically brings the ability to raise psychosocially healthy children. It is a society that takes very little account of what, in the parents' personal backgrounds, may have warped their sense of themselves and restricted their capacity to meet their children's emotional needs, or distorted their picture of how a healthy family works. It is, moreover, a society in which there is only minimal, basic consensus about what is, or is not acceptable child behavior. This often deprives parents of any feeling of community support as they try to hold their children to one set of standards while they are daily exposed, through the media and via contact with other children, to a multiplicity of differing values.

> The Tenants' Association in a small city's public housing complex may request your help with difficulties that have arisen because four young teenagers from the project have been charged with possession of drugs, and there is strong disagreement among the residents—those who are demanding that these teenagers' families be given immediate notice to vacate, and others who want to have a drug abuse information program offered in the project.
> You will need to recognize that in our society the very fact of living in a public housing project labels the residents in a derogatory way as "those Oakland Terrace people." They are defined by the rest of society as second-class citizens, and these are the feelings that they will initially bring to counseling. Also they have no way of knowing whether or not you share that discriminatory perception—unless, of course, you have worked there for some time.

The damaged self-esteem quality is absolutely critical in another way also, in that it is very often an integral part of the problem; for example, the battered wife, the school dropout, the substance-abusing individual, or the gang of "trouble makers" on the Native Reservation. In all these instances low self-esteem is a significant factor in the dysfunctional behaviors.

CLIENT NEEDS AND WORKER'S RESPONSE

Biestek presents the framework of the helping relationship as consisting of client needs and worker response in dynamic interaction (1957:17). The needs of the client must elicit from the worker an appropriate response, which is then received and responded to by the client in a manner that either shows a beginning confidence that the worker is hearing and responding to the need, or in a way that indicates that the worker has not heard them correctly. It is through this dynamic interaction that the relationship is begun and will continue to be developed.

An adaptation of Biestek's identified needs of troubled persons, with the relevant principles is set out below. These specific needs are equally relevant where the client system consists of more than one person. While the most appropriate principle is identified with each need, there is some overlap, and this will be addressed more specifically in the following chapters. The principle of responsibility for self-awareness, though related below only to certain needs where this principle is particularly necessary, must permeate the entire activity. It is the *key element of effective, truly professional work.*

The Client's Needs and the Relevant Principles

1. To be recognized as a person of worth
   - respect for innate worth and dignity of every person
2. To be cared about, attended to in a professionally responsible manner
   - the client's needs are the worker's first responsibility
3. To be confident that their secrets will be kept secret
   - confidentiality
4. To be heard with an empathic understanding of their pain
   - controlled emotional involvement
   - responsibility for self-awareness
5. To be accepted as who they are
   - acceptance
   - responsibility for self-awareness
6. Not to be judged
   - the nonjudgmental attitude
   - responsibility for self-awareness
7. To be treated as an individual, not as a "case" or a number
   - individualization

8. To be allowed to express their feelings
   • purposeful expression of feelings
   • responsibility for self-awareness
9. To be allowed to make their own choices and decisions; to retain a measure of control over their own lives
   • self-determination, which also requires:
   • active involvement of the client in the helping process
10. To be helped to take charge of their own life in more effective ways
    • empowerment
    • active involvement of the client in the helping process.
    (adapted from Biestek, 1957:17)

Each of these will be discussed in detail in the following chapters.

While virtually all troubled persons experience all these needs, regardless of their age, gender, or the kind of trouble that brings them to us, not every client or member of a client group will necessarily express them openly, and certainly not at the first contact. They may not even be aware of them as needs (Biestek, 1957:14). We shall, for example, meet some persons who initially may seem to have a need not to express feelings but rather to focus upon "practical" aspects and solutions; others may appear to hope that we can effect the work of change "on" them, so to speak, simply with their presence and passive consent.

Such needs as these may reflect a deep-seated anxiety about the process of receiving help; they may reflect hurtful previous experiences in similar situations and they can initially be blocks to getting the working relationship started.[2] Their removal will depend upon our skill and our application of the relevant principles—respect, not judging them but accepting that this is who and where they are—that is, in redirecting their approach to the helping process. The clients' beginning acceptance of such a shift will be one of the "desirable effects of a good relationship upon the client" (Biestek, 1957:18).

THE CLIENT ROLE

Although for the sake of simplicity we have been referring throughout this discussion to "the client," at first contact we actually may not have a client (Germain and Gitterman, 1980:45). We may have either an applicant, i.e., someone who has come voluntarily for help, or a candidate, someone who has come to us under some kind of external pressure to change some dysfunctional behavior. Whatever the initial mind-set of the applicant or candidate they are entitled to the full application of our professional behavior with the objective of helping them to become a client.

In my own view there are three main characteristics that will signify this shift. Several of the definitions given in the previous pages identified the purpose of social work as the bringing about of change. I consider you have a client when the person(s):

- recognize(s) a need for change;
- accept(s) you as a source of help in effecting change; and
- is/are willing to involve themselves in the helping process towards change.

I do *not* mean that we must require 100 percent recognition, acceptance, and willingness in these categories, but only a degree of each sufficient to lay a base for constructive work on the presenting problem.

> Mr. and Mrs. Boulton brought eleven-year-old Bob to Family and Children's Services at the suggestion of local police, who had recently interviewed him twice–although he had not been charged–about some vandalism around the shopping plaza near their home.
>
> I explained why I believed family therapy would be the best way to help them, and suggested a first series of three interviews with all of them present.
>
> **Mr. B:** "Well, we gotta do something to get Sergeant Majesky off the kid's back. What do you think, Mother?" (recognizing a need for change).
> **Mrs. B:** "Well, it can't do any harm to talk about it–maybe he'll listen to you; he won't to us." Bob, sitting next to his mother, rolled his eyes at his younger brother, who struggled not to dissolve in giggles. (Mrs. B seeing me as a source of help for change).

Mr. B: "Yes. Well, I thought if you'd just talk to Bob he might straighten up . . . but if you want us all here, that's how we'll try it. Okay, Mother?" (willing to involve the family in the helping process, and seeking his wife's cooperation).
Mrs. B (to Mr. B): "If you think it's best, okay." (Mrs. B will follow his lead.)

These parents may appear to have rather ambivalent motives, but we are not concerned that people in trouble come to us with high moral motivation or great clarity of aims driving them to change. In social work we are not dealing with what "ought" or "should" be, but with what is real (Biestek, 1957:72). Indeed, as someone once wrote, we need to "begin where the client is," to which someone else added "but don't leave them there" (Siporin, 1975:110).

Beginning where they are does not necessarily mean that we concur with their interpretation of the presenting problem, but only that we accept how it feels to them at this point. In such an approach, we come across as hearing what they are saying, which is a vital and sometimes underrated quality of professional social work. I say "underrated" because I believe that in beginning practice we may not realize how assiduously we need to work at hearing what people say. The quality of the helping relationship and the client's progress toward greater well-being will accurately reflect this capacity (Rogers, 1980:10, 14).

In the last example, Mr. B–clearly the spokesperson for this family–moved himself and his wife from applicants to clients during the first interview. It may take longer for Bob, or it may not. His behavior may itself be that "cry for help" that we sometimes see as the motivation behind antisocial behavior. Other applicants or candidates may take a little longer to become clients, but in my experience these three components are basic, first-step requirements for productive work toward an ultimately comfortable resolution of the presenting difficulty.

PURPOSE IN HELPING

This brings us to consideration of the *purpose* of social work. I suggest that our purpose, stated in broad terms, is threefold:

1. the resolution or at least the amelioration of the presenting problem, in such a way that:
2. the client's self-esteem is restored and/or enhanced, and
3. new tools are provided, and/or latent skills developed to facilitate more satisfying relationships and more effective problem-solving in the future.

We shall be helpful or unhelpful to those who seek, or are referred to us for service to the degree that we see our purpose and work toward its achievement in this threefold dimension. Naturally the resolution of the problem, or its amelioration, is our first consideration, but unless the self-esteem factor is kept in the forefront of all our interventions, and unless we are including a reeducation component in the work we do, the resolution of the problem will be of little real or lasting value to the client(s).[3]

The first issue to be dealt with then is the definition of the presenting problem. Clearly we and the clients initially may not be in total agreement on this. A typical example was the L. family that came to us identifying Kevin as "the problem." Although they agreed to come as a family for therapy, it seemed that they had in some measure brought Kevin in "for repairs," so to speak. The Tenants' Association in the public housing complex may see your role as adjudicating between the rival factions ("who's right?") whereas the difficulty may quite possibly have arisen at least in part from a complex set of factors that relate to a power struggle in the association itself.

As noted above, we need to start from the clients' definitions of the problem, accepting that this is how their difficulty looks and feels to them. Reaching a more workable definition together will depend on how we move toward this. If we come across as not judging the clients and respecting their right to their own perceptions, while offering a different view of their difficulties, all members of the L. family and of the Tenants' Association will find it easier to see that they all have a role in the problem's resolution. This will facilitate their beginning to work with us toward constructive change.

Many valuable books have been written in recent years on the helping relationship itself (Shulman, 1984; Ivey, 1988; Corey and

Corey, 1993, for example), and it is both unnecessary and beyond my present purpose to elaborate here. I only want to emphasize first that the relationship is built on the business that we and the client(s) have to do together. It will not be built through our knowledgeable discussion of hockey scores, or our shared enjoyment of the kitten's playfulness. I mention this because beginning practitioners have sometimes thought that discussion of the painful material of the presenting problem with the client–the nature of the probationer's crime, or the school's complaint about a child's bruises, for example–should be postponed "until I have a relationship." It is the manner in which we introduce and begin to deal with that painful material that will truly build the helping relationship. Its postponement will only increase anxiety, and quite possibly give the impression that it is something we find dreadful to talk about.[4]

Second, the quality of our helping will depend not only upon the knowledge and skill that we bring to the relationship, but upon our bringing to it that "fullness of humanity"–Biestek's beautiful phrase (1957:131)–that is the mark of what is truly professional in social work.

In the chapters that follow each principle will be discussed in detail. It will be related to the identified need of the client (person or group), with examples to show its application in work with client systems of different numerical size and interrelationships.

NOTES

1. Fried defines authority as "the ability to channel the behavior of others in the absence of the threat or use of sanctions," and power as "the ability to channel the behavior of others by the threat or use of sanctions." This enables us to see authority and power as separate but related elements (1967:10-13).

2. I have sometimes been told that making an assumption that clients have these needs at first contact is making "judgments" about them even before we meet them. We need to approach clients with an open–but not an empty–mind.

3. This is identified by Siporin (1975:48-49) as having characterized social work practice since our earliest beginnings.

4. In this connection I owe a profound debt of gratitude to J.F.B., my instructor in my second MSW practicum, who taught me that "We hurt people much more by what we don't say, than by what we do say."

REFERENCES

Biestek, Felix P. (1957). *The Casework Relationship.* Chicago, IL: Loyola University Press.

Corey, Marianne Schneider and Gerald Corey. (1993). *Becoming a Helper.* Pacific Grove, CA: Brooks-Cole.

Fried, Morton H. (1967). *The Evolution of Political Society: An Essay in Political Anthropology.* New York: Random House, pp. 10-14.

Germain, Carel B. and Alex Gitterman. (1980). *The Life Model of Social Work Practice.* New York: Columbia University Press.

Hancock, Molly R. (1986). "Authority: An Integral Part of Effective Helping." *Canadian Social Work Review,* pp. 119-132.

Hugman, Richard. (1991). *Power in Caring Professions.* London: Macmillan.

Ivey, Allen E. (1988). *Intentional Interviewing and Counselling, Second Edition.* Pacific Grove, CA: Brooks/Cole.

Rogers, Carl. (1980). "Experiences in Communication." In *A Way of Being.* Boston: Houghton-Mifflin, pp. 7-14.

Shulman, Laurence (1984). *The Skills of Helping People and Groups.* Chicago: F. E. Peacock.

Siporin, Max. (1975). *Introduction to Social Work Practice.* New York: Macmillan.

Studt, Elliott. (1954). "An Outline for Study of Social Authority Factors in Casework." *Social Casework,* 35(June):231-238. Cited in Shankar A. Yelaja, ed. (1971), *Authority and Social Work: Concept and Use.* Toronto: University Press, pp. 11-122.

———. (1959). "Worker-Client Authority Relationships in Social Work." *Social Work,* IV (January):18-28.

PART II:
THE ETHICAL PRINCIPLES

Chapter 2

Respect for Human Worth and Dignity: Social Work's Philosophical Base

The core of social work's philosophy is a profound belief in the innate worth and dignity of every human being. This conviction undergirds our Code of Ethics, and if we want to help people effectively it must permeate all our practical decisions and activities. This belief is powerfully expressed by Biestek who says that every human being

> has intrinsic value . . . [that] is not affected by personal success or failure in things physical, economic, social or anything else. (1957:73)

This concept is difficult for us, as noted earlier, because our culture has inculcated in us the idea that "respect" means "to look up to." Thus respect is commonly accorded to selected individuals, in some instances by virtue of a superior position, usually but not exclusively one of authority. Second, it is earned by superior attributes, actions or achievements.

Faced with people whose antisocial or self-defeating behavior has brought them to our service, we must not take refuge in such phrases as "there is some good in everyone" or "no one is all bad." These statements are counterfeit in terms of this principle because they show that we are still looking for what we determine are "respect-worthy" attributes. This is not a valid path to the living expression of the principle.

SEPARATING THE PERSON
FROM THE BEHAVIOR

Biestek's concept of the intrinsic value of the individual human being, unaffected by any action, attribute, or failure in or of the person, requires in the first place that we separate, conceptually, the individual self from his or her behavior. Thus we can begin to see each troubled person who comes to us not as a "child-abuser," "shoplifter," "drug addict," or "battered wife," but rather as a unique human being who is struggling with the use of antisocial and/or self-defeating behaviors as a way of coping with his or her life experiences and feelings (Biestek, 1957:73).

By means of this conceptual separation of the person from his or her behavior we can then ask what is this "innate human dignity" of the individual that this principle requires us to respect? Every person can be respected as a one-of-a-kind human being, a unique event in the whole history of the human family, one that–family resemblances notwithstanding–has never happened before and will never happen again. The belief about human dignity can be reached from many different religious, ideological, and philosophical paths. A humanistic philosophy enjoins that we must respect every human being simply because of his or her uniqueness and because he or she shares with us the human condition. Shakespeare's Richard II describes it poignantly: "[They] live with bread, like you, feel want, taste grief, need friends."

The conviction that this innate dignity and worth of the individual human being cannot in any way be diminished or lost through any deficiency, attribute, or failure in or of the person, makes it possible to respect each and every individual we meet, regardless of the circumstances in which we meet them. My respect, then, can be unwavering as I meet the physically or emotionally abusive parents, the drug-addicted teenager, the vociferous, intolerant members of the Tenants' Association, the judgmental member of the recovery group, the violent gang member, or the sexual offender (Biestek, 1957:73). Each is worthy of my respect as a person, regardless of his or her behavior.

An important aspect of this separation of self worth from his or her attributes, actions, or behavior will be our helping the clients themselves to use the concept as a means of building, restoring, or enhancing their damaged self-esteem. Our respect for them can act as a "mirror" to reflect back to them a new image—that of an innately valuable person whose dysfunctional actions do not make him or her totally unworthy. Over time, within the relationship, this respect can act as a corrective, helping to erase the self-destructive messages from their past (Middleton-Moz, 1994).

The concept of behavior as being separate from the person is constructively helpful to us in another way. Respect for the inviolate human dignity of every person does not mean that we accept and condone their behaviors; whether these are breaches of the law, ways of relating, or styles of living that are inimical to the well-being of others, of society, or of the person. We need to hold on to the distinction in our own thinking and feeling and to make it clear to the client. This will be dealt with in greater detail when the principles of acceptance and the nonjudgmental attitude are discussed. Here we need to understand that if we are to be truly helpful, our commitment to the respect principle does not give implicit approval of the clients' actions or way of social functioning (Biestek, 1957:71).

In summary, people are entitled to respect for their worth and dignity simply by right of their Being, which is totally separate from—indeed unrelated to—their pattern of thinking or acting. Our conviction about the intrinsic value of every human being will gradually enable us to make the principle of respect for their innate worth and dignity a part of ourselves, and will also enable us to express it in our practice.

THE EXPRESSION
OF THE PRINCIPLE IN PRACTICE

The persons who come to us for help with a problem almost always arrive, as has been said earlier, with damaged self-esteem. Furthermore, as already suggested, in certain instances this feeling of low self-worth may be itself a part of the cause of the problem. It is also likely that many client(s) may be unaware of this.

Most people do not think enough of themselves. We have nearly all been indoctrinated that "conceit" is unacceptable, and for some of us the alternative has been an habitual focus upon and concern about our deficiencies. Many of us have been given messages from an early age–subtle or overt and in varying degrees of severity–that we are not, and never will be good enough. Most of us long for some assurance that it is okay to be me. Even where we are reasonably successful in covering it up, we may carry with us an underlying fear of the danger that lies in being fully known to others (Biestek, 1957:75; Powell, 1969:9-12).

Thus the first need of all persons is to feel that it is safe to be themselves. Even without the pressure of needing help from a social agency, there may be a deep-seated conviction that the self is unworthy. When trouble strikes, the very existence of the problem may seem to confirm that unworthiness. Seeing themselves as being unable to resolve the difficulty by their own efforts adds more weight of evidence to the anticipated verdict of "not good enough." The old "tapes" painfully replay in their heads.

This conviction may be masked in some instances by resentment and/or anger about having been "ordered to get help," as in child neglect cases; or being placed on probation with the requirement that they change their antisocial behavior, perhaps required to attend a specific reeducation group. We need to keep in mind that this anger may be a cover-up for very real fear of possible consequences.

Our steadfast respect for our clients will need to be implicit in every aspect of our contact with them and selectively explicit at appropriate moments. It will be shown in such seemingly small matters as our punctuality for appointments and reliability about times and returning of phone calls; in promptly obtaining relevant information that we have promised (for example, the dates and times of appropriate group meetings); providing a copy of legislation pertaining to landlord and tenant; confirming linkage with home care services prior to discharge from hospital; or where and how to get low cost or free legal advice.

Even our manner of addressing the person can subtly convey whether or not we respect them. For example:

> The probation officer's report to the Court for Henrik P. states "known as 'Hank.'" As his ongoing probation officer, at my first meeting with him, I will not assume that I have the

same right that his friends and family have to call him by a nickname. I will ask him which name he prefers me to use.

Although the use of first names in most situations is now the rule rather than the exception, I will also tell him what name I would like him to use in addressing me. I believe even today this can be a dilemma for clients where, for example, there is a marked age difference between client and worker, perhaps especially where that is linked to a difference in gender. There may also be a cultural factor. I do not want to leave my client in any uncertainty about this that could add needless anxiety to the tension of our first meeting.

As outlined in the previous chapter, we shall in *all* instances be seen by our clients as persons having authority and in many as having some kind of power to affect their lives. Clients who have had unhappy experiences with previous authority figures may be very much on guard against being treated as if they were "inferior" in such situations. For some the experience of being treated with respect as persons may be totally unexpected; they may struggle to accept that it is not "phoney," and they may express this openly. We need not be disturbed by this reaction as long as within ourselves we are quite sure of our own genuineness. We also need to remind ourselves that people are not easily fooled by "phoney" civilities. These are no substitute for the quality of unfeigned respect that is the principle we are examining here (Biestek, 1957:85).

Respect Expressed Through the Other Principles

As stated earlier, our respect for our clients must permeate every facet of our work with them. It will be demonstrated by our concerned attention to their view and perception of the presenting problem. This is an indication that we recognize that each and every member of the client system—whether that be one person, a family, a formed group, or a community or organization of persons—experiences the current difficulty in ways that are unique to who they are as individuals. This is the expression of the principle of individualization (Biestek, 1957:29).

The principle of facilitating their active involvement in the helping process is of itself an expression of respect. It will give reassurance that we see our task as working with–not "on"–them. It conveys that we do not see them as totally helpless in face of the pain, personal struggle or conflict with the law that has brought them to us for service. Rather it gives a message that we see them as having capacities to share with us in the work of reaching solutions and finding new, more rewarding paths of action.

Our acknowledgement of their right to self-determination is a further expression of our respect for their right to be themselves and to retain control over their own lives. Our respect for these rights is also the basis of our recognition of their right to an assurance that their *secrets* will remain confidential and, unless the law requires otherwise, will be shared only with those others in the agency to whom we are accountable and whose help is necessary to the provision of the service (Biestek, 1957:128-132).[1]

It is our respect for them that requires us to regard their well-being as our primary responsibility, ahead of any professional or personal special interest of our own. For example, we shall not "use" them for the sake of our own professional learning, as subjects of experimental techniques in which we are less than fully qualified and/or experienced.[2] Our respect for them lays upon us the obligation to maintain a keen self-awareness, moment-to-moment, so that, for example, our own biases, hang-ups, or old fears do not get in the way of the work we must do together. This will also be a factor in our exercising controlled emotional involvement. It is important that old pain or unmet needs from our past that do not belong in the here-and-now reality–a need to be liked, or to be seen as "successful," for example–do not get in the clients' way as we share the work of achieving constructive change (Biestek, 1957:81-83).

The acknowledgement of their right to their own feelings and to the expression of those feelings is a further indication of our respect for the worth of their inner self; as is our concern to empower them where they feel a lack of their own personal or political resources. By such means clients can gain greater confidence and resourcefulness in managing their life situations more effectively in the future.

Each of the principles can thus be seen clearly as a specific expression of the cardinal principle of respect for the worth and dignity of every human being. The implementation of each in the helping process will be examined separately in the chapters that follow.

SUMMARY OF MAIN POINTS

1. The innate dignity and worth of every human being is the primary ethical principle of professional social work.
2. Individual worth and dignity is unaffected by the person's actions, attributes, or deficiencies.
3. Respect for the person can be achieved by conceptually separating the self from the behaviors and/or needs that bring them to our service.
4. Our respect can begin to have constructive effects as it addresses—implicitly and/or explicitly—the damaged self-esteem of the troubled person(s).
5. The troubled person's primary need is to be allowed to be him or herself; our respect for and acknowledgement of the worth of this self is the basis from which constructive change can begin.
6. Respect needs to be expressed in everything we say and do—and in our manner of saying and doing—throughout the helping process.
7. Each and every principle of professional social work is an expression of this core principle of professional ethics.

NOTES

1. Biestek identifies other restrictions on confidentiality that will be dealt with later in detailed discussion of this principle.
2. In certain special circumstances, with the full knowledge and consent of clients and agency, this might be acceptable.

REFERENCES

Biestek, Felix P. (1957). *The Casework Relationship*. Chicago: Loyola University Press.
Middleton-Moz, Jane. (1994). Direct communication in the course of a workshop at Sudbury, Ontario, Canada, September, 1994.
Powell, John. (1969). *Why Am I Afraid to Tell You Who I Am?* Allen, Texas: Tabor Publishing.
Shakespeare, William. (circa 1594). "Richard II," III, ii. *The Complete Works*, Peter Alexander, ed. London and Glasgow: Collins, 1951, p. 464.

Chapter 3

The Client's Well-Being: The Social Worker's Primary Responsibility

The second ethical principle of social work is that the clients' interests are our primary concern and first professional responsibility. The well-being of the clients must never be secondary to any interests of the worker.

The NASW Code of Ethics introduces this principle with the statement that our primary professional responsibility is to

> serve clients with devotion, loyalty, determination and the maximum application of professional skill and competence. (NASW, 1993, II, F.2:5)

The elements that are integral to the implementation of this principle, as identified in the NASW Code, encompass the following strictures:

> Exploitation of the relationship by the worker for personal advantage is totally contrary to this principle. (NASW, 1993, II, F.2:5)

*   *   *

Jim, an MSW worker with six years experience, had recently moved from a family service agency into a clinical private practice with three partners. His background was entirely in family, couple, and individual therapy. Practice in this partnership was based on each worker counseling independently, with opportunity for peer consultation, but no regular supervision.

Jim learned that Karen, one of the partners in the practice, was specializing in family mediation with separating and divorcing couples, and he became interested in this area of work. He suggested to Karen that he would like to accept couples for mediation and would discuss these cases with her as he went along. He felt it would be a good way to "learn on the job."

His partner pointed out to Jim that this would be totally unethical. Mediation requires specialized training. Jim could not ethically present himself to clients as offering a service in which he had neither training nor experience. The NASW Code demands that the worker "not misrepresent professional qualifications, education, experience, or affiliations" (1993, I, B.2:3). To "use" such clients as a means of learning mediation skills would be a flagrant breach of his professional commitment of placing his clients' rights to service before his own desire–commendable as it might be–to learn a new area of practice.

This example highlights the issue of competence, which is central to the implementation of this principle. In its section on Competence and Professional Development, the NASW Code states that the social worker has an obligation to "become and remain proficient in professional practice and the performance of professional functions" (NASW, 1993, I, B:3).

We can only maintain our competence by not becoming complacent in the level of our work, and by being attentive to new developments in professional thinking and method. We have an obligation to our clients to acquire new knowledge, and to rethink our practice in the light of new concepts introduced through professional reading and attendance at seminars. The CASW Code is explicit that:

> the social worker shall have, maintain and endeavour periodically to update an acceptable level of knowledge and skills to meet standards of practice of the profession. (CASW, 1994, 3.6:12)

Most employers encourage professional staff to attend workshops pertinent to their area of practice, and in some instances provide an annual training budget for this purpose. Current budget restrictions, however, are forcing employers to find more economical training programs.

Adequate competence, however, is not only a matter of knowledge and skill. Our state of physical and mental health can be a significant factor affecting the quality of our practice. Both the NASW and CASW Codes cite this as part of our responsibility for maintaining competence in order to serve the clients' interests. The NASW Code states that:

> the social worker whose personal problems, psychosocial distress, substance abuse, or mental health difficulties interfere with professional judgment and performance should immediately seek consultation and take appropriate remedial action by seeking professional help, making adjustments in workload, terminating practice, or taking any other steps necessary to protect clients and others. (NASW, 1993, I, B.4:3)

Sometimes the effect of such conditions–substance abuse, depression, personal problems–may first be identified by a supervisor. We may have been trying to cope and/or deny the effect such struggles might be having on our practice, depending on our level of self-awareness. Corey and Corey state that

> Mental-health professionals who themselves are in the midst of a psychological morass and who are still attempting to carry on their normal client caseloads are breaching a basic ethical code that states that the welfare of the client is supreme. (1993:198)

Self-awareness is a value principle expected of the professional social worker, and is dealt with in detail in the following section. Here it needs to be stressed as integral to our responsibility for competence in its widest sense. The critical factor in providing effective service to our clients is a constant watchfulness about the condition of the self-as-instrument in the professional relationship.

Personal difficulties arising from the work situation itself can have a negative impact on our service. We may, for example, find one member of a couple in marriage counseling uncongenial. For a worker of either gender, this could be a matter of gender and/or power issues. A male worker may find an authoritarian husband threatening, because of negative childhood familial patterns; or he may find a meek, submissive male partner irritating for similar reasons. Male or female workers may also find a dominant, powerful woman threatening, perhaps triggering childhood memories of their parents' marriage.

Similarly, female workers with a strong feminist philosophy may initially find it difficult to maintain a balance between the rights of each partner in a marital struggle. They may find themselves rejecting the assertive husband or the meek, submissive wife. The emotions triggered may be from their feminist bias, or from familial background carryover.

Whatever the reason for such difficulties, we need to recognize that they are affecting our service to our clients. These difficulties may come across clearly in recording, and the subject may be raised by a supervisor. A consultation with the supervisor can enable us to perceive just what is happening, and to correct it. If the problem cannot be resolved by these means, transferring the case to another worker may be appropriate. Pain from our childhood must not be allowed to get in the way of service to our clients (Corey and Corey, 1993:195-199).

Sometimes in such cases the client who feels he or she is being discriminated against is strong enough to complain and ask for a transfer. When this does not occur, or when worker and client cannot resolve the issue, the worker must give the client a rational and respectful reason for the transfer. The CASW Code states that:

> A social worker shall immediately inform the client of any factor, condition, or pressure that affects the social worker's ability to perform an acceptable level of service. (CASW, 1994, 1.4:10)

In a note to this section, which defines "condition" similarly to the NASW code section cited earlier the CASW Code suggests that "A disclosure under this section may be of a general nature" (1994, 1.4: 10, note #10). Thus it would be ethical for a worker who was going into a program for alcoholism to state simply "a health problem" as the reason for a transfer of clients.

Another example of meeting this obligation ethically could be the following:

> Randy, a student-intern in fieldwork placement would not necessarily have to be specific about the reason for suggesting a transfer or referral for a family with whom he was working. He would not need to state that Mr. J's manner in family interaction—even his appearance—had triggered troubling emotions from his relationship with his own domineering, rejecting father and that these were blocking his ability to be objectively helpful. He could simply say that it had been agreed between him and his supervisor that a more experienced worker could help the family better than he can.

The worker must not act in any way that is based on discrimination against clients on any grounds whatsoever. (NASW, 1993, II, F.3:5)

The NASW Code specifically identifies matters of race, color, sex, sexual orientation, age, religion, national origin, marital status, political belief, mental or physical handicap, or any other preference or personal characteristic, condition or status. (NASW, 1993, II, F.3:5)

Most of us have prejudices or biases, some of which we may know and acknowledge and others of which we may be unaware. We may need help to become aware of these, so that they do not interfere with our respect for each and every client. This is essential in our accepting fully our responsibility to provide them with effective service.

Some of our prejudices are very subtle, which makes them hard to face and identify. For one worker it may be an unspoken but pervasive rejection of obese persons; for another it may be a bias against people who habitually use profane or vulgar language. These are idiosyncratic biases that have no place in the helping relationship.

> Lorraine Bogart came to a family counseling center asking for help with a "personal problem." Anita, the worker on Intake, learned that one year ago Lorraine aged 24, had left her husband. They had been married for three years and had no

children. There had been a lot of conflict throughout the marriage. More than once since separating, Lorraine had begun to find herself attracted to other women. She remembered feeling this way occasionally during high school, and had found it disturbing, but she had decided these feelings were just "school-girl crushes" and tried not pay any further attention to them. She had always felt "shy and awkward" around boys and had not dated in high school. Ken, her husband, was the first man she had dated, and they married after knowing each other about two months.

Recently she had met a young woman, five years older than she, who told her she was lesbian, and that she would like to get to know Lorraine. Lorraine was feeling very confused. She found herself strongly attracted to this woman and wanted help in sorting out her feelings about whether or not she was in fact lesbian. She was concerned about what that could mean for her, her family, and her job at a bank.

Anita was very uncomfortable as Lorraine shared her difficulty. As far as she knew, she had only once before met a lesbian woman, a classmate at college. Homophobia had been discussed during her college courses, but her strong disapproval of homosexuality on moral grounds had prevented her from doing any reading or taking part in discussion, in or outside of class.

Although Anita knew that two of her colleagues, one male and one female, counseled homosexuals with problems, she found herself reluctant to assure Lorraine that the agency could help her. She told her that a worker would get back to her about an appointment. She then kept putting off recording the Intake interview for processing by the Intake assignment supervisor. Doing this would necessitate discussing Lorraine's struggle about her sexuality with the supervisor, and Anita knew she would find this very difficult.

The result was that Lorraine's request for help went to the "bottom of the heap" on Anita's desk, and was not processed until some time had elapsed, well beyond the requisite number of days that was the rule between Intake, consultation, and assignment to a worker. When the Intake supervisor discussed this delay with Anita, she recognized that her homophobia had blocked Lorraine's access to the help that she needed. Furthermore, when the worker to whom the case was assigned called Lorraine to make an appointment, she said she had changed her mind about getting counseling. It is quite possible that Lorraine had interpreted the lengthy delay as confirmation of the rejection she anticipated as she struggled with redefining her sexuality.

The supervisor discussed homosexuality and her homophobia with Anita, and recommended some reading and discussion with a more experienced colleague to help her prevent this from affecting service for another client.

Discussion

This worker's inability to recognize and immediately discuss her homophobia with a supervisor, so that the referral could be appropriately processed within a reasonable time, is a clear breach of the principle under discussion here. The worker's prejudice impeded the client's receiving the help she sought and to which she was entitled.

BOUNDARIES OF THE PROFESSIONAL RELATIONSHIP

Workers must refrain from any dual relationships with clients or former clients. (NASW, 1993, II, F.4:5)

We need to establish "clear, appropriate and culturally sensitive boundaries for the helping relationship" (NASW, 1993, II, F.4:5). It is unethical for us to act in any way that confuses the clients about the nature of this relationship, its purpose, and its boundaries. Such clarity helps to ensure that our shared objectives can be achieved.

In the first place the relationship is not a reciprocal one. As will be discussed in subsequent chapters, we need to be aware of our responsibility to meet the needs of the client and not our own. The only need of our own that we can legitimately seek to meet is that of satisfaction in giving the best of our knowledge, skills, and caring concern to each client.

Second, the relationship is structured in terms of our use of time. Only so much of our time can be allocated to each case situation. In assessing this allocation we need to take into account all the individual factors in each situation, but some limitation is a reality for us and for our clients.

Agencies vary in the expectations of or restrictions they place upon staff about giving their home phone numbers to clients; this will vary according to the clientele served by the agency and the agency's provision for emergency response. It may, however, be left to the worker's discretion in particular cases, taking into account the clients' life situation and emotional state. In my own experience in child welfare and in a general family service caseload, clients have very rarely abused this. I recall a depressed client telling a colleague in family service that just having her number and knowing that she could call, had given her the security she needed to keep her going between sessions.

Third, it is confusing and counterproductive for clients if we become too "social" in the helping relationship. For example, if visits to the client's home are part of the process, we need to be careful that we and the clients understand that these have a specific purpose, so that the work for planned change is not clouded by too much "sociability."

Fourth, the roles of worker and client must not be confused by the introduction of a relationship that is unrelated to the shared tasks of the helping process.

David had worked with the K family for four months. They had focused on the K's marital problems, which were exacerbated by Mr. K's poor work record. This poor record was mainly caused by his inability to control his temper when he was required to accept instructions from superiors. The marital therapy had relieved much of their difficulty, and both partners had felt more secure in their relationship at termination of service. Mr. K had begun to look at his difficulty in accepting direction at work. However, three months later he had still not been able to find a job and had phoned David feeling quite down about this.

David felt it would be empowering for Mr. K to fix D's car. Mr. K's work on the car proved unsatisfactory, and David struggled with finding the best way to explain this to Mr. K.

Discussion

David's supervisor discussed with him how his shifting the base of the relationship from worker-client to customer/service-provider had produced confusing feelings for both parties. It set Mr. K up for another work failure, but what was even more damaging was that it had placed him in a one-down position with David, one of the very few persons in his life whose respect for him had not depended on his meeting any "performance" requirements.

Social workers are strongly advised not to counsel either members of their own family or persons with whom they have been friends prior to the request for help. The worker's objectivity–critical for the accurate assessment of the clients' problems and their behavioral responses to those problems–cannot be maintained where previous close relationships exist. Pope comments that

> When counselors engage in dual relationships, they tend to impair their professional judgment, the danger of exploiting the client increases, and clients are put in a vulnerable position by the power implicit in the therapist's role. (1985)

We must recognize the risks for the client if we move toward a friendship role during the provision of service. Perhaps this client is a professional person; you share the same philosophy of life, sense of humor, and some particular interest–books or theater, for example. Corey and Corey point out that this dilemma is not easy to resolve. They suggest that if such a situation arises, we need to examine our own motivation and that of our client, and to assess as honestly as possible how this may affect our ability to be effectively helpful (1993:325).

> Sexual activities with clients are prohibited under any circumstances. (NASW, 1993, II, F.5:5)

This is very clearly a breach of the professional relationship's boundaries. It constitutes a use of the client for the worker's own gratification, sometimes—sad to say—under the guise of being part of "treatment." In most professional jurisdictions workers would lose their license or certification to continue practice if such an accusation were proved against them.

If a worker finds him or herself physically attracted to a client he or she has an obligation immediately to discuss this with his or her supervisor or consultant. It is essential for beginning workers to have the opportunity to explore such a dilemma in a nonthreatening atmosphere. Pope and Vasquez state that

> to feel attraction to a client is not unethical; to acknowledge and address the attraction promptly, carefully and adequately is an important ethical responsibility. (1991:107)

Where a worker feels that the client is attempting to attract him or her physically, the first step would be to discuss this openly with the client, stating the inappropriateness of this behavior in the professional relationship. If this was not accepted by the client, and/or not followed by more appropriate behavior, the worker would be justified in offering either a transfer to another staff member or terminating service.

This would need to be done in a calm, nonpunitive way, simply emphasizing the inappropriateness of this behavior in a professional helping relationship. This is one example of the "precipitous termination" of service that is further discussed below. Corey and Corey discuss these issues extensively (1993:327-328).

PRACTICE OBLIGATIONS

> Accurate, clear information must be provided to the clients about the extent and nature of the service available, and of their risks, rights, and obligations associated with the service provided. (NASW, 1993, II, F.6:5)

This is a significant reflection of our respect for all those who come for help, whether they come voluntarily or are involuntary candidates for service under some external mandate, such as probation or child welfare law. It is a recognition of every potential client's right to be fully informed about the service and how it will be provided. Clients need to know what they can expect from us as workers and what is expected of them in accepting the conditions established by agency mandate and policies, or the stipulations of any court order.

In family counseling, as has been stated earlier, whole family sessions are routinely a condition of giving service. In adoption services, attendance at group meetings is usually a requirement of the study and assessment process. The obligation to clarify the service process applies equally to staff in public agencies and in private practice where fees are charged.

Where a worker is committed to a particular school of practice, thought, and intervention method, the client has the right to be given a clear understanding of this, how it will be used, and what it may involve. Levy warns that such an exclusive identification

> . . . may prove a possible deprivation to a client if the social worker's commitment to it results in a failure to avail the client of the benefits of another mode or regimen of service. (1976:136)

In some agencies, workers would be free to transfer the client to another worker whose mode of service would be more attuned to the client's needs. If it is agency policy to adhere to one model of practice, it would be necessary to offer an unwilling client other resources in the community that could better meet their needs. Whether or not agencies have the right to limit their service to one school of practice—and thus restrict their staff—is a matter for discussion, but cannot be addressed here.

With full and clear information, voluntary applicants can make a realistic decision about whether or not they want the service being offered. Involuntary candidates have the security of knowing what is involved for them as they move into the process of changing the circumstances and/or actions that have brought them under a legal mandate.

Other Client Rights

The clients' rights and obligations are fairly clear: the right to be a partner in determining the goals of change and to being fully informed of the methods employed; the right to confidentiality; the right to regularly scheduled sessions with the same worker, of a specified length, and at fairly short intervals; the right to the worker's undivided attention during each session; and the right for the sessions to continue over a period of time mutually agreed upon. This last may vary with agency policies. In some instances there is a stipulated number of sessions for preliminary assessment, with a further period being negotiated for the resolution of the presenting problem(s). These rights overlap with the obligations the client assumes in accepting the worker-client contract, which may be either written or verbal.

The risks for the client are more complex. When fees for service are paid we need to discuss the financial cost in the beginning and from time to time thereafter. If any form of hypnosis is to be part of therapy clients need to realize that they may discover things they would rather not have known. This would be part of ensuring they can make an informed choice about such a course of therapy. Other risks may be incurred as they make changes in thinking, feeling, and acting, which affect personal, work, or social situations. These may be significant in clinical practice but may also be very relevant in work with groups, communities, and organizations. With any size client system, we need to discuss such risks in the course of achieving the objectives of professional intervention.

When individuals, couples, or family groups are offered participation in a group as part of therapy, we need to discuss very clearly with them how such a group usually functions and what is expected of participants. In order to make an informed choice of whether or not such a form of therapy is suitable for them, it is important that clients understand that questions of trust, confidentiality, and sharing will arise, and that the group may make rules of participation for themselves.

> Social workers are required to seek appropriate advice and consultation from superiors in the interests of providing effective service. (NASW, 1993, II, F.8:5)

This is a part of our ethical obligation to provide to all clients the best possible service that we and the agency can offer. The need for supervisory consultation must be clearly understood by all staff as being first, an appropriate way of sharing the responsibility for meeting this obligation, and second, a way to improve one's practice strengths and work on areas of difficulty. It is a particularly important part of fieldwork internship. Consultation is an integral part of our ethical responsibility for providing the best service we can. Experienced workers need not perceive it as a reflection on their ability.

In most agencies a regular time for supervision is provided for all professional staff. In many instances this is done one-on-one by a senior staff member appointed as supervisor. In some cases, where selected groups of staff are considered to have attained a certain level of competence, supervision may be offered in regularly scheduled peer consultation, in small groups, with or without a supervisor present. Workers in private practice are also expected to consult with a qualified colleague, either a practice partner or someone outside the practice, on a regular basis or as the need arises.

TERMINATION OF SERVICE

Service must be terminated when it no longer serves the clients' interests. (NASW, 1993, II, F.9:5)

There are basically four kinds of termination of professional service. The first is usually called "natural" termination. This occurs when both client and worker agree that the goals have been met, or at least have been achieved as far as possible. Second, there is the "preset" termination, where the period of intervention is determined by a court order, or is set by a mutually agreed upon contract between client and worker.

Third, there are "forced" terminations. These occur when, for whatever reason, the time of termination is set by administrative circumstances, over which the client has no control. Examples are when a client—adult, adolescent, or younger child—is discharged from a residential treatment setting or when the worker leaves the agency for some reason. Termination of service provided by fieldwork interns belongs in this category. An important consideration in all forced terminations is whether or not the service is to be continued after the worker or student intern leaves.

Lastly there are "unplanned" terminations, where a client "drifts away" during the course of therapy by breaking contact in some way. Each type is included in the discussion that follows.

Termination of service, for any reason, is an important event for clients and workers. The reason for termination and the manner in which it is carried out will have significant meaning for each individual, family, or group with whom we are involved. Some of these meanings all clients will share; others will give rise to highly individual reactions (Hellenbrand, 1987:765). All will require our careful consideration.

Preset Terminations

The period of time during which service is offered to clients is variously determined. For involuntary candidates–in probation and child welfare services, for example–there is often a legally mandated period of time during which service must be provided. The objective here is that the required changes in behavior or lifestyle will be brought about within that period. The termination date is thus known by both parties from the beginning and is integral to the service plan.

Where the application for service is voluntary, and in child protection service where parents accept the agency's intervention without a court order, it is customary now for workers and clients to enter into some form of contract. This may be either verbal or written, outlining the expectations on both sides, the number and spacing of the sessions, and the period of time estimated as necessary. This might be an estimate of the time required for completion of the process of change, or a target date at which to review progress and to look at setting up a further service plan.

Whether the service is provided to voluntary clients or involuntary candidates, this mode of practice is valuable for both clients and workers as a means of stimulating motivation and purposeful work on both sides. Gould's study of MSW student interns found that students who did not tell clients at the outset of the relationship that their time of working with them was limited by their student status "did not set clear-cut goals with their patients" (1978:266). Gould further suggests that setting goals and time limits may become more generally the norm in that

. . . with increasing demands on available mental health resources and requirements for accountability of treatment, it seems necessary to set goals and to establish criteria for termination. (1987:266)

This is the usual practice in group work where a group has been set up specifically for persons sharing certain difficulties–behavior control, anger management, or eating disorders, for example–or other kinds of struggles that impede their healthy functioning. Hellenbrand reminds us that for group members termination means a twofold loss. They are losing the close and trusting association with group members with whom they have shared an intimate experience, as well as the relationship with the worker (1987:768). Where this sense of loss is expressed by clients–openly or covertly–it needs to be addressed as part of the termination process. This will be discussed in more detail in examining forced termination.

Natural Termination

The ethical obligation to terminate service and the professional relationship when there is no longer any need for it would seem to be obvious. However, as noted above, terminating service has meanings for worker and client that may get in the way of a satisfactory ending. Hellenbrand points out that for workers there are emotional struggles that may impede an objective decision to terminate. These include "worker satisfaction, disappointment or guilt about what has or has not been accomplished" (1987:65).

Hellenbrand suggests that natural termination needs to be recognized by the client as "graduation." Recognition must be given for what has been achieved and for the hard work this has taken; the new tools and skills for living, now being used, need to be identified, and reenforcement should be given for specific instances of their successful use (1987:765-767). The clients need to be reassured that we no longer believe they need our help in sustaining these gains. In helping them to accept the end of a meaningful relationship, Fox, Nelson, and Bolman quote Blanchard (1946) who says that

it is sad to say goodbye to someone who has been loved for a while and to whom one feels grateful, but it is a satisfaction to become independent of help and be freed from the obligation to keep appointments that sometimes interfere with other interests. . . . (1969:56)

In other instances we have to accept that some of our clients cannot attain the level of change that we wanted for them, and that we initially believed they could reach. We must accept that they have achieved as much of the desired change as they are able to handle–or perhaps willing to attain. This is often difficult for us, because we want the best for our clients.

We may need to recognize and accept our deficits as part of the situation's reality. It is possible, too, that these clients may come back at some future time to seek help with the unfinished business that we can see still remains. If they do come back, we need to be careful not to perceive it as failure–on our part or theirs.[1]

Lastly, in some cases where we feel we have been ineffective, we may try to postpone formal termination, hoping–against the evidence–that, given more time, we can do a better job. In all such situations our ethical obligation dictates that we terminate the service, recognizing that these clients will not benefit from any further interventions on our part. Supervisory consultation will help us to learn from such cases, and to eliminate an unrealistic guilt load.

Forced Termination

Fox, Nelson, and Bolman (1969); Northen (1982); Bolen (1972); and Hellenbrand (1972) suggest that if the relationship has been one of trust, unwavering acceptance of the person(s), and genuine caring for their feelings, ending the relationship may trigger the old pain of previous losses in some of our clients. For them, the relationship may have been the first in which they felt truly valued and cared about as a person in their own right.

Bolen's (1972) discussion[2] suggests that this may be particularly true for adolescents being discharged from residential care. These factors, while common to all terminations, are perhaps particularly significant in forced terminations.

Whatever the reason for ending the contact, the client should be informed well in advance of the pending termination whenever possible (Fox, Nelson, and Bolman, 1969; Gould, 1978; Bolen, 1992). The NASW Code formalizes this, stating that

> Clients must be notified promptly when termination or interruption of service is anticipated, and appropriate transfer, referral or continuation of service must be arranged, taking the clients' needs and preferences into account. (1993, II, F.11:6)

This is a pertinent reality for fieldwork interns. The student needs to inform clients well in advance of the date on which they will be completing their assignment. Gould's study of MSW students in fieldwork states that

> Students who told patients the duration of their fieldwork *at the beginning* [found that] they and their patients seemed to perceive termination more as a growth experience than as a trauma. (1978:266, emphasis added)

Transfer to Another Worker

Some clients will need to be transferred to other workers for ongoing service. Here the worker or student will need to clarify, in consultation with his or her supervisor or field instructor what the client's needs are, and to take their preferences into account. This could involve a particular need or preference as to gender, religious affiliation, or the language in which the service is being offered.[3]

Some ground is nearly always temporarily lost for clients when there must be a change of workers. Careful "matching," wherever possible, can minimize this setback, and the manner in which the transfer is carried out is important. If at all possible, the new worker needs to be introduced to the client by the student or worker who is leaving the case (Mumma, 1989:24). If this is done effectively, clients who have developed a secure trusting relationship with the student can see that these two workers respect each other and that "their" worker has confidence in this new person. I believe this is important in giving some reassurance to the client. This plan is not always possible where there is a change of staff. A lack of agency resources may necessitate a gap in service. We need to recognize with the client that this makes the transfer even more difficult.

Workers coming into this transfer situation need to be comfortable with the likelihood that the clients may refer to their former worker with affection and a sense of loss, sometimes even with a seemingly exaggerated tribute to his or her fine qualities. We need not interpret this as implying that we are "not as good as" Carl or Lois. It is simply an expression of the client's feelings of loss of someone who was important to them. If we knew and admired the former worker as a colleague, we can join the clients in agreement with such compliments. If we did not know the previous worker, or we knew him or her but didn't share the client's admiration, we can voice our recognition of how much the relationship has clearly meant to them.

Clients who greet a new worker as a welcome change from a previous one with whom they did not get along present a different challenge.[4] Many of us have been greeted with such statements as "Gary just never understood my problem" or "Melanie made it tough for me because she always took the kids' side." These statements may simply indicate that they didn't "click" with their former worker. It may or may not reflect anything real about that worker's ability. It may also be an expression of anger about the former worker's "desertion" that they dared not—or had no opportunity to—express to him or her.

Unplanned Terminations

As mentioned earlier, unplanned terminations occur when clients terminate of their own accord, indirectly, by not showing up for scheduled appointments and not calling to reschedule. We need to address this directly (Hellenbrand, 1987:767). In my opinion, this is best done by a letter from worker to client, recognizing that they have decided not to continue, and assuring them that they will be seen if they ever decide to seek help again. I believe that doing this by letter puts them under less direct pressure than a phone call. Hellenbrand suggests that if we ignore the clients' "no-show" they may have the feeling of "having been cast as 'truant,' [which] may make it difficult for [them] to return" (1987:767).

> Services must be withdrawn precipitously only in exceptional circumstances; in doing so workers must take all circum-

stances into account in order to minimize adverse effects. (NASW, 1993, II, F.10:5)

One instance of precipitous withdrawal of service in exceptional circumstances is cited above, in the case of the client seen by the worker as trying to be sexually seductive. Other instances can occur, such as the sudden onset of serious illness or sudden death of the worker. At the time of this writing, agency staff downsizing in many regions is increasing the frequency of transfers and–most regrettably–terminations. This adds to the urgency of our attention to all the factors discussed above in helping clients deal with these experiences constructively in order to minimize potential harm as much as possible.

Professional ethics demand that we assess each and every action we take, from the inception of service through termination, against the measuring rod of the clients' best interests.

SUMMARY OF MAIN POINTS

1. A cardinal ethical principle for social workers is that in our every professional undertaking, the best interests of the client are our prime concern.
2. We must not exploit the helping relationship in any way for our own advantage.
3. The clients' best interests demand that we continually work to maintain and enhance our professional competence.
4. This will require vigilant self-awareness about our biases, and a nondefensive response when we are shown by others that these are impeding our giving effective service.
5. It will also demand that we readily become aware, or accept help in becoming aware, when our physical or psychological health is impaired in ways that affect our practice.
6. Our effectiveness can be impaired by our having or developing feelings about a client's personality traits that we find difficult to accept. We must accept appropriate help in dealing with these feelings, or accept and assist in a transfer to another worker.

7. We need to establish and maintain appropriate boundaries of the helping relationship. Dual relationships are invariably damaging to clients.
9. We cannot counsel relatives or close friends. It is impossible in such cases for us to maintain the objectivity that is essential for effective helping.
10. Sexual activities with clients are absolutely prohibited.
11. All clients must be fully informed about the nature of the service and how it will be offered.
12. Terminating service, regardless of the reason, requires our concerned attention to its meaning for each client or group of clients. The termination process must be carefully worked out so that it is a positive experience for all—those we have not helped as well as those we have.

NOTES

1. I believe it was Carl Rogers who said that no one ever conducted the perfect interview.

2. Bolen's article is important reading for students interested in or already working with youngsters in residential settings.

3. The CASW Code includes as an obligation in observing the primacy of clients' best interests, offering service where possible, in the language chosen by the clients (1994, 1, Section 1.7:10).

4. Nobly restraining your urge to say "Yeah, I know what you mean, I couldn't stand him either."

REFERENCES

Blanchard, Phyllis. (1940). In *Psychiatric Interviews with Children*. New York: Commonwealth Fund. Cited in Fox, Nelson, and Bolman (1969).

Bolen, Jane K. (1972). "Easing the Pain of Termination for Adolescents." *Social Casework*, 53(9):519-27.

Canadian Association of Social Workers. (1994). *Social Work Code of Ethics*. Ottawa: Canadian Association of Social Workers.

Corey, Marianne Schneider and Gerald Corey. (1993). *Becoming a Helper, Second Edition*. Pacific Grove, CA: Brooks/Cole Publishing Co.

Fox, Evelyn F., Marian A. Nelson, and William M. Bolman. (1969). "The Termination Process: A Neglected Dimension in Social Work." *Social Work*, 14(4):53-63.

Gould, Robert P. (1978). "Students Experiences with the Termination Phase of Individual Treatment." *Social Work* 48(3):235-269.

Hellenbrand Shirley C. (1987). "Termination in Direct Practice." In *Encyclopedia of Social Work*, 18th Edition, Vol II. Silver Spring, MD: National Association of Social Workers, 765-770.

Levy, Charles S. (1976). *Social Work Ethics*. New York: Human Sciences Press.

Mumma, Edward W. (1989). "Reform at the Local Level: Virginia Beach Empowers Both Clients and Workers," *Public Welfare* 47(2): 15-24.

National Association of Social Workers. (1993). *NASW Code of Ethics*. Washington, DC: National Association of Social Workers.

Northen, Helen. (1982). *Clinical Social Work*. New York: Columbia University Press, pp. 279-299. Brooks/Cole Inc.

Pope, Kenneth S. (1985). "Dual Relationships: A Violation of Ethical, Legal, and Clinical Standards," *California State Psychologist* 20:3-5. Cited in Corey, Marianne Schneider and Gerald Corey. (1990). *Becoming a Helper, First Edition*. Pacific Grove, CA: Brooks/Cole Publishing Co.

Pope, Kenneth S. and Melba J.T. Vasquez. (1991). *Ethics in Psychotherapy and Counseling: A Practical Guide for Psychologists*. San Francisco: Jossey Bass. Cited in Corey, Marianne Schneider and Gerald Corey. (1993). *Becoming a Helper, Second Edition*. Pacific Grove, CA: Brooks/Cole Publishing Co.

Chapter 4

Confidentiality:
The Essential Component
of Professional Helping

DEFINITION OF CONFIDENTIALITY

This is a central principle of professional social work's code of ethics, one of the most significant elements of the helping relationship. Albers and Morris deem it "equal in importance or more important than other practice issues" (1990:11-26). Levy says that it is the prerequisite of clients entering into a helping relationship, and that without it no effective service can be offered or received (1976: 51-52).

Current developments in social work practice have influenced both the ethical and practical demands upon workers in meeting this obligation. This chapter discusses these issues, dilemmas, and demands.

Confidentiality is defined by Biestek in the following terms:

> Confidentiality is the preservation of secret information concerning the client which is disclosed in the [course of the] professional relationship. Confidentiality is based upon a basic right of the client; it is an ethical obligation of the social worker, and is necessary for effective social work service. The client's right, however, is not absolute. Moreover, the client's secret is often shared with other professional persons within the agency and in other agencies; the obligation then binds all equally. (Biestek, 1957:121)

Social work service, in order to bring about change, is virtually conditional upon the clients' sharing with us personal and private information about themselves and their life situation. This is stated by Albers and Morris:

> Social work is unlike other professions in that its prime and often only instrument of change is the information bound within the professional relationship itself. (1990:11)

THE CLIENTS' NEED

The primary need of clients in disclosing their trouble is not to be judged. People are understandably reluctant to share private information that may put them or their past decisions in a bad light. This anxiety about being judged–perhaps as incompetent, even culpable–is often quite realistic, having been confirmed by previous experiences of opening up to others.

We must make it clear from the outset that the facts and feelings clients disclose throughout the contact will not become public knowledge, and that they will always be informed about who else needs to learn about their trouble and for what purpose.

Some clients will have more difficulty than others in trusting our integrity in these matters. We need to recognize and accept their difficulty explicitly, without becoming defensive. Our scrupulous attention to honesty and a nonjudgmental attitude in all our contacts will gradually reassure them that their trust is not misplaced.

ETHICAL OBLIGATIONS
AND PRACTICE ISSUES

Professional codes of ethics provide injunctions and guidelines for practitioners in the implementing of this principle in practice. Agencies also have responsibility to develop policies and guidelines for staff that fit their mandate and their administrative system's framework (Biestek, 1957:126, 131; CASW Code, 1994, 5.2:14). Social workers must be completely familiar with their professional

Code of Ethics; they need to be fully informed about the policies and procedural guidelines set out by their employers and to know the legal requirements of the jurisdiction in which they practice.

The NASW Code of Ethics (1993, II, H:6 provides instructive guidelines for social workers, stating that

> The social worker should respect the privacy of clients and hold in confidence all information obtained in the course of professional service.

1. The social worker should share with others confidences revealed by clients, without their consent, *only for compelling professional reasons.* (emphasis added)
2. The social worker should inform clients fully about the limits of confidentiality in a given situation, the purposes for which the information is obtained, and how it may be used.
3. The social worker should afford clients reasonable access to any official social work records concerning them.
4. When providing clients with access to records, the social worker should take due care to protect the confidences of others contained in those records.
5. The social worker should obtain informed consent of clients before taping, recording, or permitting third-party observation of their activities. (NASW, II, H:6)

The Right to and Limits on Confidentiality

The first and second statements deal with the right to and the limits on confidentiality. Watkins (1989) cites Jagim, Wittman, and Noll (1978) in identifying two types of confidentiality–absolute and relative–the latter being the most common in social work practice. Jagim, Wittman, and Noll describe the situation of absolute confidentiality, which in their view could only be very rarely given, as:

> the ethical position which demands that the therapist would never break confidentiality under any circumstances. [This refers to information that] the therapist would never share with anyone else; put in any written form, e.g., case record, feed into a computer, or discuss orally. (1978:459)

Before giving this level of assurance to a client, the worker would need to be absolutely certain that the client's expressed demand in requiring such secrecy could in no circumstance be overridden by other requirements such as those cited by Biestek:

- the law, [which can vary from one state or province to another],
- the rights of other persons, and
- the rightful good of society as a whole. (1957:123)

Therefore, we usually can offer clients only relative confidentiality, acknowledging that information can be shared with others under certain circumstances (Watkins, 1989:133).

General Legal Limits, and the Tarasoff Decision

Any professional person learning of the abuse of a child in the course of his or her professional activity, usually has a legal duty to report such knowledge to the child welfare authorities. In many jurisdictions any citizen has an obligation to report information that could prevent a crime, but a therapist has a special "duty to report."

This was established in case law in 1974 in California with the decision in the landmark case of *Tarasoff vs. Regents of University of California.* At the first hearings of this case, the Supreme Court of California "imposed liability on the therapists because of their failure to warn the murder victim of their patient's threat to kill her" (Kopels and Doner Kagle, 1993:101). In the course of further hearings in 1976, the court changed the clause of "duty to warn" to a "duty to protect intended victims from the violent acts of the therapist's patient" and further concluded that:

> public policy favoring the protection of the confidential character of patient-psychotherapist communications must yield to the extent to which disclosure is essential to avert danger to others, [and that] the protective privilege ends where the public peril begins. (Kopels and Doner Kagle, 1993:102-103)

The Canadian Association of Social Workers' Code of Ethics (1994) identifies this as an ethical obligation and specifically refers to the client's family and *Tarasoff* in this connection, and states that:

A social worker shall disclose information acquired from one client to a member of the client's family where

(a) the information involves a threat of harm to self or others,
(b) the information was acquired from a child of tender years and the social worker determines that its disclosure is in the best interests of the child. (CASW, 5, 5.25:16)

The NASW Code guidelines leave this matter at the very general level of "compelling professional reasons" while the CASW Code attempts greater specificity.

Subpoena of Worker and Record

In child protection and child custody matters, or the corrections field, the court may subpoena the worker and the record. The client needs to understand that in such a situation neither we nor they have any choice about full disclosure. In some jurisdictions social workers have legal privilege in court, in that they are not required by the Court to divulge information given to them in confidence. However, these are exceptions and normally the client must be told that legal privilege does not apply to the social worker.

LIMITS WITHIN THE AGENCY

Clients must be informed clearly and explicitly from the outset that there are limits on confidentiality within the agency. Their personal information cannot be strictly "between you and me." We must inform the client that our notes or tape recordings of case records have to be transcribed by a secretary; that our sessions with them must be open for consultation with a supervisor and/or in some agencies a peer team group; and that sharing at both these levels is an essential element in providing them with effective service. In fee-for-service agencies a bookkeeper and/or accountant will have access to their name and the status of their account. Albers and Morris cite a study showing that providing this information to the client does not affect the client's willingness to disclose their problems fully (1990:11).

Clients will need explicit reassurance that agency policy binds all persons within the agency who have access to the records to the same commitment to protect their confidentiality (Biestek, 1957:125).

Computerized systems of case recordings raise many complex questions. Generally it can be said that rigorous safeguards against unauthorized access to or theft of computer records must be a top priority for agencies.

The question of who needs to know the clients' private information, however, brings up the matter of staff coffee room chat. While discussion there with a co-worker is often simply a reflection of our interest in our work, to discuss a client with a worker from another team or department who has no responsibility in the case is a breach of the confidentiality that we have guaranteed to our client (CASW, 1994, 5.19: 16; Whittington, 1988:95-96).

Confidentiality and Agency Public Relations

The function of confidentiality is to protect the client, *not the agency*. It must not be used to protect the agency from external evaluation. Most agencies have policies and procedures setting out who may and who may not talk to the media. This may arise, for example, when a dissatisfied client "goes public" with his or her complaint. Some agencies have learned—at a price—that citing "confidentiality" as the reason for "no comment" can sometimes be interpreted by the public as a "cover-up." These are judgment calls that must be decided at management level.

Contact with Other Agencies

Instances often arise where effective service requires that another agency must be contacted and relevant information shared. It is essential that clients first know precisely why this is necessary, and second, that they know as exactly as possible what information is to be shared. A signed form consenting to the release of information must be obtained from the client in all cases. This form should define the purpose of the sharing and what is to be shared and should state a time limit beyond which it will not be valid (Whittington, 1988:95). These are the essential elements of what is known as "informed consent." Similarly, if another agency or service requests information from us about our clients, we must maintain confidentiality until we receive from that agency a consent–signed by the client and witnessed–for us to release information to the agency person(s) involved.

In small communities, where informality among professional colleagues may be customary, we must guard carefully against breaches of professional ethics in this matter. We must not permit ourselves to lapse into informal exchanges of information that may come perilously close to "gossip." We always need to obtain written consent to the release of any and all information (Whittington, 1988:95).

THE AGENCY RECORD

The question of what is recorded is a difficult issue and is subject to debate in the profession. The first issue is the ethical aspect of how the information concerning the clients' difficulties is obtained.

The CASW Code (1994) gives the guiding principle about how information is obtained as:

> clients shall be the initial or primary source of information about themselves and their problems unless the client is incapable or unwilling to give information or when corroborative reporting is required. (1994, 5.4:14)

Many child welfare and children's mental health situations require corroborative reporting. For example, a school or medical record may be necessary to assess the difficulty and to initiate an appropriate intervention plan. In the field of corrections–probation or parole, for example–corroborative reporting also may be essential.

In cases where clients refuse consent for us to obtain information from an outside source, we must explain to them fully the possible consequences–legal and/or personal. This is another instance of our obligation to help clients make a fully informed decision.

Regarding what is recorded, it is now generally agreed that the official record of the agency needs to contain strictly factual information relevant to the clients' problem and its resolution, the professional assessment, and the intervention plan. The initial assessment may require amendments as things progress and change, and the effectiveness of the intervention plan requires monitoring as it moves toward the resolution of the presenting difficulties (Wilson, 1978:218). Workers are urged now to be cautious and absolutely explicit when recording statements of professional opinion. As the CASW Code states:

> The social worker shall not record in a client's file any characterization that is not based on clinical assessment or fact. (1994, 5.5:11)

The following provides a practice context for some of the above cautions and requirements.

As a worker in a child welfare agency in a rural area, you receive a referral from the school in late November, expressing concern about ten-year-old Melissa Keppel's daydreaming at school, tasks not accomplished on time, and her general appearance of being "sad and withdrawn." This seems a sudden change for this child, who last year was an A student in all her studies and a normally happy little girl around the school.

The referral comes by phone from the school nurse, who explains she is speaking for Melissa's classroom teacher, with the principal's knowledge and approval. The nurse has tried to talk to Melissa, but the child just clammed up and said "nothing was wrong." The school has attempted to contact the parents, but has received no response to phone messages or a letter expressing their concern and asking for a meeting. The nurse says you are free to explain to Melissa's parents that the school has asked you to contact them.

Your first contact is with the parents in their home, having arranged a convenient time with Mrs. K by phone beforehand. You observe that she is naturally nervous and defensive at your visit. (So many families have heard that a visit by the child welfare agency worker is but a prelude to speedy removal of the children, court hearings, etc.) She says the school is making a fuss over nothing. "It's just a phase she's going through," Mrs. K says. When you try to arrange a time when she and her husband will both be at home, Mrs. K is very vague and evasive about her husband's working hours and how the meeting can be arranged.

You explain to Mrs. K that it is the agency's legal responsibility to investigate such referrals with the objective of helping the family and finding out what is troubling Melissa. You also explain that you, or an agency colleague, would be working with them to help them give Melissa the kind of help she needs to be happier and to do as well in school as she used to do.

In response to your question about any changes in the summer that might have affected Melissa, Mrs. K says that the only change was that in July she went back to work as an RNA at the local hospital. She now works steadily two weeks on days and two weeks on night duty. When she works at night, her husband baby-sits Melissa and their six-year-old son, except when his lodge nights—twice a month—fall in those weeks. Then the teenage daughter of a neighbor watches Melissa. Mrs. K says rather defensively that when her husband is home in the evening with the children he "might have a friend or two in for a beer to watch a hockey game now and then."

This contact raises some speculations. Is there a possibility that Melissa is experimenting with drugs? Do they feel confident in the responsible behavior of their young neighbor? Does Mr. K drink excessively with "a friend or two" when he is baby-sitting, to the extent that Melissa is frightened by their noisy behavior? Is it possible that her father is sexually abusing her or her little brother when her mother is at work?

In consultation with your supervisor you realize that it would be premature to raise any of these questions with Mrs. K at this point. You will therefore begin—as always—with the terms of the referral, which in this case are the school's expressed concerns.

You will need to explain to Mrs. K that it is necessary for you to talk with Melissa's classroom teacher, the principal, and the school nurse, and you will suggest that it is important that she and her husband, or at least one of them, should be there. You may offer to drive her to the school if transportation is a problem during her husband's working hours.

You will need to make it clear to Mrs. K that it is to their advantage to cooperate with you and the school. To refuse to do so could possibly leave them open to being judged as uncaring about Melissa's welfare. You will need to discuss this when Mr. K can also be present, so that together they can make an informed decision about whether or not to cooperate.

Discussion

The Keppel family's confidentiality can be protected at this point by simply informing the school nurse that you have visited the family and that you plan to arrange a meeting with both parents and the concerned individuals at the school as soon as possible. It may require tact, but it is important that you do not get into any further conversation with the school nurse or anyone at the school at this time. To do so would be a serious breach of confidentiality.

You and your supervisor agree that it would be inappropriate to make an appointment to talk to Melissa at school at this point. In order to help this child effectively, your priority is to enlist the parents' cooperation.

Most school district authorities have policies in place about whether or not you may interview a student at school without one of the parents present. There is also an ethical issue: most child welfare agencies feel that to interview the child at school is the same as interviewing an adult at their workplace. The child must be called out of the classroom, and is thus singled out among her classmates, exposing her to their questions later. This verges upon a breach of confidentiality for your clients–this child and her family. In some cases it may be necessary, but the pros and cons always need to be carefully weighed. In general it is best not to obtain information from the child without the parents' knowledge unless you believe a separate interview is essential.

Other Exceptions

The CASW Code gives a directive where information is required from other sources, stating that the social worker

(a) shall explain the requirement to the client, and
(b) shall attempt to involve the client in selecting the sources to be used. (CASW, 1994, 5.7:14)

The Keppel family is an example. Another example might be a medical report to support an application for worker's compensation as the result of an injury at work. Another could be the need to obtain a health history of birth parents from a child welfare agency; adopted adults may need this because of health problems that have arisen for them or their child.

The question of how we maintain confidentiality in family therapy, group work, and community practice has only fairly recently come to professional attention. Some issues that arise in family therapy will be discussed under protecting the privacy of others when allowing access to the record. Confidentiality in group work and community practice will be addressed in the section on multiclient systems.

Reasonable Access to Agency Records

NASW's third statement reads

> The social worker should afford clients reasonable access to any official social work records concerning them. (1993, II, H:6)

This raises first the question of what is recorded, and second, how to define "reasonable access." The first is in part governed by the professional Codes of Ethics, and also by each agency's statements of policy in this matter. The second, unless it is within circumstances governed by statute, has to be—within the framework of the agency's statement of policy—virtually a judgment of the worker and his or her superiors. The specific aspects of the case where this arises will need be taken into account in making such decisions.

It is currently general policy that the record's contents need to be clearly discussed with clients. There must be no "surprises" for the client on seeing the record, or hearing the worker give evidence from it in court.

In terms of what is "reasonable access," as a general principle, the CASW Code states that

> 5.14. A social worker is obliged to follow the provision of a statute that allows access to records by clients.

5.15. The social worker shall respect the client's right of access to a client record subject to the social worker's right to refuse access for just and reasonable cause.

5.16. Where a social worker refuses a client the right to access a file or part of a file, the social worker shall advise the client of the right to request a review of the decision in accordance with the relevant statute, workplace policy or other relevant procedure. (1994, 5:15)

Reasonable access will thus be a matter of whatever law is in force in the local jurisdiction, or of agency policy. Again, this may include the possibility of individual decisions in certain cases where exceptional circumstances arise.

Protecting the Privacy of Others when Allowing Access

NASW's fourth statement stipulates that when clients are given access to their record, workers have a responsibility to protect the confidence of others contained in those records. (1993, II, H.4:6)

This can arise particularly in practice with couples and families. While the majority of sessions are held with both partners of a couple, or all members of a family, some members may be seen individually for certain purposes of their own in the course of the work. This is done only by agreement with all members of the client system receiving service. In family therapy, for example, the children may be seen at a certain point in sibling pairs, the entire family may be seen as a group, or the parents as a couple. Information may be given to us in the course of such sessions that one member may request be kept confidential from the partner, or from the other family members. We are obligated to protect the privacy of that individual, exactly as we would in one-to-one relationships.

Of course, in the interests of the therapeutic plan, such a request will need to be discussed with the individual in terms of the actual purpose of their guarding the secret from the other(s), of the function of such secrecy, and the potentially constructive or damaging result to the relationship of full sharing. But if such discussion does not alter the individual's position then their privacy must be protected. How this is done will depend upon the agency's policy, which sets out how records are maintained. For example, records of sessions with individual family members, or with the children's group, may be maintained separate from—although kept with—the family therapy record.

This respect for individual choice will also apply in cases where one member of the client system wishes to give consent to release information to a third party, but another member or members refuse. These persons have the same right to protection of their confidential information as those in an individual service relationship. Thus the consent to release will apply only to the information given by the individual signing the consent.

The question of confidentiality in working with groups and in community practice will be given detailed attention in the section on multiclient systems.

SHARING OF SESSIONS WITH OTHERS

NASW's fifth guideline concerns the sharing of a session with other persons, within or outside the agency, by means of direct observation, taping, or videotaping. (1993, II, H.5:6)

Informed consent is a requirement in all such instances. We must ensure that the client(s) clearly understand with whom this record will be shared and for precisely what purpose. A written consent must be signed by all members of the client system who will be present. The consent must state the specific purpose of the video, the date of the proposed taping, and the date when it is to be shown. The purpose is usually educational.

For example: From time to time during a student's practicum, selected sessions conducted by the student may be videotaped in order that the student and his or her field instructor may evaluate the student's progress in interviewing skills, etc.

In some agencies it is customary for each member of a team periodically to conduct an interview while the supervisor and team members observe from behind a one-way screen. The purpose again is primarily educational—to assist beginning practitioners, and often to also evaluate experienced team members, or to assist them with blocks that may have arisen in their practice.

There may be other educational uses: an experienced practitioner or teacher may want to use such videotapes in whole or in part to illustrate specific points of instruction when offering a professional workshop or seminar.

MULTICLIENT SYSTEMS

Several authors (Moore-Kirkland and Vice Ivey, Thomas, and Dolgoff and Skolnik, among others) have made significant contributions to current thinking about how systems theory has impacted our overall approach to therapeutic intervention, whether with individuals, whole families, groups, or in community practice. These writers' examples, particularly but not exclusively from work in rural communities, provide a convincing systems theory basis for reconsideration of practice applications of the confidentiality principle.

Working with Groups

Dolgoff and Skolnik affirm that in group work

> The multiple clients involved necessitate that special attention be given to establishing confidentiality as a group norm for each member, for the group as a whole and the worker. (1992:106)

The CASW Code states as follows:

> The social worker in practice with groups and communities shall notify the participants of the likelihood that aspects of their private lives may be revealed in the course of their work together, and therefore require a commitment from each member to respect the privileged and confidential nature of their communication between and among members of the client group. (1994, 5.23:16)

This will mean that the worker must clearly set the situation out at the first meeting, and give a reminder from time to time thereafter, especially following any meeting at which particularly sensitive revelations have been made by one or more members. It will be necessary at the same time to explain fully to the group the limitations that are placed upon confidentiality by the law and the rights of others. The question of what limits might be applicable in any group will depend, in part, upon the group's composition and purpose, and the legal requirements in the local jurisdiction.

Group work is used for many purposes in social work today. Groups may be formed for growth and development, such as Adult Children of Alcoholics or Adult Survivors of Childhood Sexual Abuse. Others may have the objective of changing antisocial or criminal behavior, such as anger management groups, groups for physically abusive spouses or parents, shoplifters, or drunk driving offenders on probation.

In any such groups, Dolgoff and Skolnik suggest that

> the supportive atmosphere and spirit of mutual aid engendered in effective group work practice might result in revelations regarding situations such as the abuse of a child, the intent to harm someone, the abrogation of a parole or probation agreement. (1992:106)

Here again it will be essential that the worker is fully informed about his or her professional obligation, under the law, to disclose information received in the course of professional activity, and that he or she makes this completely clear to the group members, at the outset and from time to time as work goes on.

Other groups are often formed with the objective of imparting essential knowledge about a particular issue or process. The focus may be either on dealing with a specific problem, or helping people engage themselves in a particular service that they are requesting. Groups may be formed in a children's mental health center for parents of children diagnosed with attention deficit disorder. Family counseling agencies sometimes form groups for parents bereaved by sudden infant death syndrome. It is now customary for adoptive applicants to be required to attend group meetings as part of the adoptive process. This is virtually routine regardless of the specifics of the application–age, gender, ethnic origin of the child requested, the couple's stated acceptance of physical or developmental handicap, and so on.

In all or any of these groups, the feeling of safety within the group facilitated by the effective group worker may, as Dolgoff and Skolnik point out, bring about disclosure of very painful experiences or events, or of actions about which an individual may have carried unresolved shame–perhaps initially valid or unrealistically self-imposed–for a long time. As stated above it will be vitally important that the confidentiality of the sessions is made a part of the contract that is entered into by the group at its first meeting, and that reminders are given at subsequent meetings.

Rural Environment: Special Factors

Moore-Kirkland and Vice Ivey provide a solid theoretical and ethical base for their contention that practice in a rural environment creates a need for reappraisal of our traditional ways of honoring confidentiality. As noted above, they view this as essential, whether we are working with individuals or multiclient systems. They base this stance on the principles of systems theory stating that it has

> provided an integrated framework for viewing change in the interactions among various parts of social systems . . . and given more attention to changing relationships among and between systems. (1981:319)

The social context in rural areas has a degree of intimacy that does not exist in large cities. These authors discuss the effect on daily living of families having lived in the same area for several generations; of everyone knowing virtually everyone else, and of the interrelatedness of families; of the immense amount of everyone's business that is known by their neighbors, the extended family, and those with whom everyone does essential business. They cite, for example, alcoholism, wife and child abuse (1981:320). One could add poor money management, the inability to hold a steady job, and an apparent lack of ambition in looking for work. Any of these behaviors can effectively define individuals and families in the eyes of those among whom they live, especially in the kind of close quarters that characterize the rural setting.

Thomas says that the community is going to involve itself one way or another in what it sees as some solution to the presenting problem(s). He suggests that secrecy, in the name of professional confidentiality, only serves to feed "an aura of secrecy and shame which evolves into gossip." This is clearly counterproductive in helping the client (1976:19). This author states further that

> Inherently built into the structure of small communities is a great potential for intervention that is often neglected: *network forces*. (1976:19, emphasis added)

He illustrates what support can be marshalled for a woman coming out of the hospital after treatment for mental illness. He involved a representative group of women in the community in looking at the client's need for acceptance and the enlisting of supportive, friendly help as she reintegrated back into her home community (1976:19-20).

This example highlights not only the difficulty but the actual ineffectiveness of attempting to maintain a traditional approach to confidentiality in this kind of setting.

Moore-Kirkland and Vice Ivey raise three basic questions about holding to traditional patterns in the rural environment. These are:

(i) Is it feasible?
(ii) Is it effective?
(iii) What about ethics?

The small community characteristics noted above do not only apply in rural areas. They also characterize to somewhat the same extent the social context of a small low-rental housing complex in a small city. The following example illustrates the three-point focus given above in such a setting.

> You are a social worker for the local housing administration. Mr. Juarani approached you three months ago about his wife's drinking and its effect on the children. Mrs. J was quite abusive when you visited her at home, and she refused to become

involved. The couple have four children ranging in age from seven to fifteen years. Mr. J appreciated your concern but felt there was no more you could do. He found it hard to deal with his older children's resentment that he would not just take them and leave Mrs. J. They didn't understand how he could still care about their mother when she was so uncaring about him and them.

Three weeks later Mrs. J had been drinking at home in the afternoon and took the car to buy some groceries. She was involved in an accident at the mall, barely managing to avoid hitting a small child who had wandered into the parking lot as she drove in—much too fast—from the street. Only the mother's presence of mind and swift action saved the child from being seriously injured (the child only suffered bruises and brush-burns). Mrs. J then careened into a light pole and another car, and someone called the police.

As a result of this, Mrs. J was charged with driving while ability impaired, her licence was suspended, and she was placed on probation. A condition of her probation was that she attend an addiction program daily at a center located near where she lived and on a bus route.

Mrs. J was much shaken by this accident. The child's size, hair color, and jacket had, for an instant, looked like her own son at the same age. The idea that she had nearly killed her son Jason haunted her. However, she did not attend the addiction program daily. She skipped several sessions and showed up intoxicated one time.

Mrs. J asked about a one-month residential program she had heard about; she felt that it would give her the consistent support and protection she needed to make a really good start on her sobriety. Her probation officer and you agreed. She seemed highly motivated, was admitted, and did, in fact, get a firm hold on the program there.

The question now is how to provide effective help to the Juarani family as Mrs. J, apparently fully committed to sobriety, returns to them and to the housing project community. You have worked in this community for three years and have been involved in some projects of the Tenants' Association that showed their strong wish to be thought "decent and respect-able"—not to be looked down upon by the rest of the Project population. The Juaranis are one of a minority of Hispanic immi-grant families in the mainly black population of the Project.

Discussion

This brings up the first of Moore-Kirkland and Vice Ivey's ques-tions. Is it feasible to protect this family's confidentiality when a fairly large proportion of their neighbors and acquaintances are fully aware of Mrs. J's alcoholism, her charge, probation terms, and resi-dential treatment?

Their second question is whether or not it is going to be effective to work with the Juarani family as if their social relationships were not an integral part of their daily lives, both as individual members in their respective age groups and as a family? Moore-Kirkland and Vice Ivey say that this is not constructively helpful, and they cite Speck and Atneave who say that

> to act as if ignorant of the client's inter-relationships in the community is to be naive about the very social relationships that may be a source of difficulty for the client. (1973:154)

The third question raises the ethical issue of whether or not to maintain the traditional pattern of client family confidentiality as strictly in this particular setting. Moore-Kirkland and Vice Ivey contend that the knowledge base of systems theory is the deciding factor here. Systems theory has taught us that change in any part of the system brings about—because it necessitates—change in other parts of the system and thus of the system itself. These authors ask:

> knowing this, is it ethical to work exclusively with one mem-ber [I would add "or a subsystem"] of a social system, while consciously excluding from the process of change those who will also be affected? (1981:321)

Speck and Atneave state that maintaining confidentiality in the traditional sense in the small community setting can actually be harmful, in that a pathological social network owes most of its rigidity and inflexibility to the presence of secrets, collusion and alliances, which must be broken up if change is to occur. (1973:154-155)

With the Juarani family, you will need to attend first to the necessary shifts in relationships within the family brought about by Mrs. J's sobriety, and second, to reintegrating the family, with a sober Mrs. J, into the Housing Project community. Regarding family relationships, it is very likely that Mr. J and the older children have, so to speak, learned to "work around" Mrs. J, virtually excluding her from the family's domestic organization and planning. Her attempts to break into this pattern, during temporary sober periods while she was still drinking, have likely been the cause of fights and distress and were most likely resolved by another lapse into drinking by Mrs. J. This family now needs to shift its organizational and relationship patterns to accommodate Mrs. J as a participating member, asking her to have a voice in the family's choices and decisions.

Viewing the Juarani family as a subsystem of the Housing Project, we can also recognize that the same kind of shift in relationships will be a factor in this relatively close-knit community. It will be important for Mrs. J that friends, acquaintances, and neighbors come to accept the new, sober Mrs. J, including her as a full participant in Project activities. Biases, prejudice, and ignorance will probably be factors to be recognized and dealt with in this process.

In this connection, Moore-Kirkland and Vice Ivey describe the case of a man returning home from psychiatric treatment as

a social event, not a private affair. The question is not whether the community knows about the problem but what blend of information and disinformation has evolved. Speculation will fill in the gaps. (1981:320)

With the Juarani family then, it will be both ethical and effective for you to discuss with and obtain the family's agreement for some work with their friends, closer neighbors, and acquaintances, providing education about alcoholism and some sharing of Mrs. J's feelings about her drinking and newfound sobriety. Her AA sponsor, or another AA representative, could be helpful at such gatherings. With your help as facilitator, support can be enlisted for Mrs. J, such that she and her family can feel comfortably welcomed back into their community as fully participating members.

In their listing of guidelines, the same authors support such a plan in stating that it helps

> family, neighborhood, and community to develop new ways of dealing with each of its parts on a realistic basis. (1981:321)

In this way we can realize "our professional commitment to promote optimal social functioning between people and their environments" (Moore-Kirkland and Vice Ivey, 1981:320).

SUMMARY OF MAIN POINTS

1. Confidentiality is central to the helping relationship, and the clients' trust in its maintenance is essential if effective service is to be provided. Confidentiality in professional practice is governed by the Codes of Ethics.
2. The clients' anxiety about divulging private information must be recognized as real and valid.
3. Confidentiality is limited by the agency's structure and policies, the law, and the rights of others. We need to be clear and explicit with clients about these limits.
4. Social workers need to be fully informed about the policies of the agency which employs them and about the law in the jurisdiction where they work.
5. Where information is to be shared, both agency and client need the protection of a signed consent form describing the information to be shared and the purpose, and stating a time limit on the specific consent.
6. Clients are to be the main source of information about themselves and their trouble.
7. Agency policy will determine what information about the clients' difficulties and the progress of work is recorded, in what form, and in how much detail.
8. Everything that goes into the record is discussed with the client(s).

9. Any videotaping or audiotaping of a session with a single client or with a multiclient system, must only be done with a written consent, signed by all members of the client system involved.

10. Systems theory suggests that complete confidentiality for the individual may need to be varied in practice so that intervention to promote constructive change can be truly effective with families, groups, and communities.

REFERENCES

Albers, Dale A. and Richard J. Morris. (1990). "Confidentiality." *Canadian Social Work Review* :11-26.

Biestek, Felix P. (1957). *The Casework Relationship*. Chicago, IL: Loyola University Press, pp. 120-133.

Canadian Association of Social Workers. (1994). *Code of Ethics*. Ottawa, Canada: CASW, Chapter 5, pp. 14-19.

Dolgoff, Ralph and Louise Skolnik. (1992). "Ethical Decision-making; the NASW Code of Ethics and Group Work Practice: Beginning Explorations." *Social Work With Groups*, 15(4):99-112.

Jagim, Ryan D., William D. Wittman, and John O. Noll. (1978). "Mental Health Professionals' Attitudes Towards Confidentiality, Privilege, and Third-Party Disclosure." *Professional Psychology*, 9:458-466.

Kopels, Sandra and Jill Doner Kagle. (1993). "Do Social Workers Have a Duty to Warn?" *Social Service Review*, 67(1):101-126.

Levy, Charles S. (1976). *Social Work Ethics*. New York: Human Sciences Press, pp. 51-54, 141-142.

Moore-Kirkland, Janet and Karen Vice Ivey. (1981). "A Re-Appraisal of Confidentiality." *Social Work*, 26(4):318-322.

National Association of Social Workers. (1993). *Code of Ethics*. Washington, DC: NASW, Section H, p. 6.

Speck, Ross V. and Carolyn Atneave. (1973). *Family Networks*. New York: Random House, pp. 154-155.

Thomas, Noel. (1976). "Network Intervention in the Small Town." *Human Services in the Rural Environment*, 1(July):19-22.

Watkins, Sally A. (1989). "Confidentiality and Privileged Communications: Legal Dilemma for Family Therapists." *Social Work*, 34(2):133-136.

Whittington, Ronaele. (1989). "Button Your Lips." *Journal of Independent Social Work*, 3(2):93-100.

Wilson, Suanna J. (1978). *Confidentiality: Issues and Principles*. New York: The Free Press, p. 218.

PART III:
PRINCIPLES REQUIRED OF THE WORKER IN THE PROFESSIONAL USE OF SELF

Chapter 5

Responsibility for Self-Awareness: The Self as Instrument in Helping

Responsibility for self-awareness is a key principle of our profession. Because professional helping is a system of dynamic, immediate interaction between persons, self-awareness is considered the critical attribute required of the helper for effective practice. Cournoyer states that

> Social Work is a professional practice involving the conscious and deliberate use of self. The social worker's self is the medium through which knowledge, attitudes and skill are conveyed. (1991:10)

Combs, Avila, and Purkey, in identifying what they call the "self as instrument" concept, state that:

> Effective operation in the helping professions is a question of the use of the helper's self, the peculiar way in which he is able to combine his knowledge and understanding with his own unique ways of putting it into operation to be helpful to others. (1973:5)

If this instrument is to be effective, we must maintain it, as we do any other tool, at its maximum efficiency.

> The human instrument requires continuous checking and calibration. [Unlike most physical instruments] human organisms

tend to become increasingly sharper, stronger and more effective with use. . . . the self can be made an ever more effective
and sensitive instrument with exercise and discipline. (Combs,
Avila, and Purkey: 201)

The method of "honing" our instrument for maximum effectiveness is the cultivation of self-awareness.

Cournoyer states that "self-understanding is a lifelong process"
(1991:10). Becoming a professional helper demands that we frequently reassess ourselves as thinking, feeling, and acting persons in
our relationship to others. The depth and intensity of this undertaking will be new for many students. As we learn professional practice
skills we need to make a habit of checking the moment-to-moment
reality of our inner thoughts and feelings (Lammert, 1986:376).
This is essential to ensure that our perception of what is being said
or expressed by the client is not distorted by our unrecognized
personal biases. That can lead to an unhelpful response that does not
meet the client's immediate need because it is unrelated to his or her
here-and-now reality. When such inappropriate responses do occur,
we need to examine just where they come from, and why at that
particular point in a session. This will be discussed in more detail
later.

Thinking, feeling, acting, and social aspects of the self can be
expressed and examined under the headings of beliefs, opinions,
and values. These influence our feelings about ourselves and our
way of relating to our social environment. Second, we can examine
the self in terms of our self-perception, which includes self-esteem
and our patterns of response to persons and events that may trigger
"old" psychosocial reactions that do not relate to the immediate
reality. Lastly we can look at how we relate to others from the
framework of our own personal needs.

There is much overlap between these areas and all, to a greater or
lesser degree, influence how we feel about ourselves. All are ingredients of who we are and how we relate to others. Our perception of
self and our behavior are the product of how we have learned to deal
with all our life experiences up to that point in time, in our family, at
school, at work, and in social contacts. Failing to understand who
we are may well impede our helping efforts.

BELIEFS, OPINIONS, AND VALUES

Early in our professional education we are introduced to detailed information about North American society, including its political and legal structures and economic organization. The preconceptions and judgments that we bring to this experience will be a function of our ethnicity, the socioeconomic standing of our family of origin, and/or, in the case of mature students, the status we have achieved prior to coming to a school of social work. It may also reflect the political convictions and affiliation of our parents, which we may have either adopted as our own or rejected in favor of different–perhaps opposing–views transmitted by other role models. Cournoyer calls this our "social context" (1991:17).

Some of the sociopolitical and socioeconomic information offered in the beginning courses may in fact be new to us, or it may be presented in a manner and from a value base that is more or less unfamiliar. This may challenge beliefs and opinions that we have held quite firmly until this time, and that–up to now–we have found worked satisfactorily. Not only are we asked to reexamine these beliefs and opinions, but as we proceed into specific professional courses, classroom discussion will require us to review them in the light of the values of professional social work, with the objective of making those values our own.

Some students have more difficulty than others with these areas as they begin their professional education. Many of us are taken by surprise by an unexamined prejudice; for example, when we first encounter–as a classmate, instructor, or client–a member of a different, perhaps adversely categorized, ethnic or socioeconomic group, or a homosexual. We can also be caught unawares in beginning fieldwork, as noted earlier, when our professional ethics require that we respect persons whose behavior–homosexuality, for example–violates a previously unquestioned conviction about right and wrong behavior.

These beliefs and opinions can influence our response to many kinds of antisocial behavior, and even to questions of unemployment and social assistance. They can be obstacles to overcome as we begin to take on responsibility for the objective assessment of the needs and rights of people in trouble.

Kevin, a white, middle-class student, twenty-one years old, had always believed that the majority of people on social assistance, especially single mothers, had chosen to let the taxpayers support them rather than get out and get a job. He thought that they had an easy time of it, and that most had TV's, smoked, and drank beer—all at the taxpayers' expense.

Kevin had never questioned this belief because he had heard it from his father and mother ever since he could remember, and until he came to university he had only met one person who thought differently—a young minister, temporarily in charge at the family's church. Many of the predominantly middle-class, suburban congregation disapproved of his so-called "radical"—some said "socialist"—views, and were relieved when he left to go to an inner city ministry.

Kevin's motivation to become a social worker stemmed from getting to know his father's younger brother, recently returned home because of failing health, from a long career as an agricultural advisor with the UN in the Third World. Kevin admired his uncle and enjoyed talking to him and his aunt, a nurse, about the work they had done. It troubled him that his uncle and his father, a successful businessman, did not get along. His father felt UN money was being wasted on such projects.

His uncle's obvious respect and compassion for the different kinds of people with whom he had worked had not challenged Kevin's basic views about poor people here at home. The Third World people were clearly "different" people, he thought, from an alien cultural, political, and economic background.

At college, Kevin found that many of his classmates had very different views from his own about poor people, unemployment, and alcohol and drug abusers. Moreover these "liberal" views were promulgated by some of his professors, even the white, obviously middle-class ones. Visiting lecturers who worked in social agencies talked about their clients in ways that reminded Kevin of his uncle's attitudes.

A field visit to a public housing community center introduced him, face-to-face for the first time, to a group of mothers on welfare. These women were working on a grant proposal to raise funds to organize a toy library and indoor play space for their younger children. They talked about how they felt when their older children came home from school crying because they were labelled "those Ridgeview Park kids" and of not being able to afford the things for their children that would help them feel "less put down" at school. They spoke of hopes and dreams for a better future for their children. In the journal report required by the instructor after this visit Kevin wrote that these women "talked as if they really cared about their children."

For the first time Kevin began to see poor people as troubled human beings, struggling with tough circumstances and with feelings about the way those circumstances affected their lives. His experience of meeting others–his instructors and his peers who held different convictions about people living in poverty– shook his previously unexamined convictions. The direct contact with the women at the community center forced him to stop categorizing people on welfare–"those welfare bums"–and he began to think about them in more directly individual ways.

Discussion

With the help of his course instructor, Kevin, who was not an insensitive person, learned two important things about becoming a professional helper. First, he realized that his previous attitudes were simply the result of his ignorance of the reality of poverty. They were merely mistaken beliefs, and did not make him a "bad person." Second, he found that he could change them in the light of new information and thus grow as a person who genuinely wanted to help people in trouble. This was this student's first encounter with the concept of "self-acceptance" an important aspect of the helper's self-esteem (Combs, Avila, and Purkey: 297; Bate, 1968:94-95). This will be discussed in more detail later.

SELF-PERCEPTION

Our self-perception is a function of our early psychosocial development in our family of origin (Cournoyer, 1991:10) and the influence of persons and events throughout our lives up to now. It is a combination of our level of self-esteem, our perception of our responsibility toward others, and of the expectations that we have of others in relation to our own self-worth. Each of us grew up in a family within which there were certain rules, spoken or unspoken, about such things as the expression of anger, sadness, fear, and joy. Furthermore, in the family of origin each member may have adopted and consistently played out a certain role. Cournoyer cites as examples the family rescuer, scapegoat, peacemaker, hero, enabler, parental child (1991:11). I would add "comedian."

Something in the professional helping situation may trigger an habitual reaction in us–coming out of our particular family experience–and we may automatically respond in a way that is inappropriate to the clients' need. This can take us by surprise because until we begin to examine our feelings and responses in the immediate helping situation we are often not conscious of such reactions as part of our behavioral repertoire. Cournoyer points out that

> ... sometimes it is entirely proper for a social worker to use a part of his family-based self in social work practice. However, the professional social worker should be aware that he is doing so. (1991:11)

It is this habitually knowing what we are doing, moment-to-moment, that constitutes self-awareness for the social worker.

> In her first fieldwork placement, Mary-Lynne recorded that one of her beginning sessions in marriage counseling had "gone well" because the couple had "stopped quarreling" and "Mrs. K sat quietly without interrupting her husband while he talked about his unhappiness in the relationship." At the same time, this pattern showed up in Mary-Lynne's work with another couple. Mary-Lynne's field instructor asked her to look at whether or not this was really helping these couples find a different way to resolve their differences.
>
> It became clear that Mary-Lynne was overconcerned with the couples' "quarreling," particularly because it seemed to her that both wives "went on and on in a loud, complaining voice." She believed that nothing constructive could be

achieved unless the other partner was "given the floor." Mary-Lynne was very upset when at the end of their third session Mrs. K told her that she felt Mary-Lynne "never wants to hear my side of the story, you only ever listen to Dan."

With the help of her field instructor, Mary-Lynne realized that she was repeating a pattern of role-behavior established in her family from a fairly early age. The middle child, and only girl in a family of three siblings, she was very conscious of being her father's favorite, and of her mother's consistent rejection. Her parents' relationship was conflicted. While quite young Mary-Lynne observed that her mother frequently nagged and criticized her father at great length. He usually remained silent for some time until he would suddenly explode into a verbally violent rage. Dreadful, long, drawn-out, shouting uproars between the couple would follow.

While her older brother just took off at such times, either to his room or outside, her younger brother was terrified, and hid under the stairs. At about eight years old, Mary-Lynne found that if she could get her father's attention with anything before the explosion—a broken roller skate, a homework problem, a question about sports, (like her father, she followed professional sports)—her father's outburst often would not happen. She was able to do this, in spite of her mother's rebukes, because her father would pay more attention to her while obviously ignoring his wife's complaints. When Mary-Lynne was successful—as she often was—her mother would simply give up her tirade and leave the scene. Thus a distressing major row was avoided.

Mary-Lynne had cast herself as the family "peacemaker" and had persisted in this maneuver until she left home for college.

Discussion

In discussion with her field instructor, Mary-Lynne was able to see that she was reacting to the possibility of the K's "quarreling" in much the same way that she had with her parents. She was able to express how much their "quarreling" disturbed her. It had triggered the old fear of parental uproar from her childhood and she had felt it was effective to "stop" them.

She understood that effective marriage counseling did involve intervening when an argument between the couple was clearly going nowhere, and helping them take time out to look at their ways of resolving disputes. However, she had not been aware that her manner of "stopping the quarrel" was at the expense of Mrs. K She was repeating her effective childhood maneuver—"forestalling a row."

As with the student in the previous example, Mary-Lynne was able to see that by becoming aware of the roots of this inappropriate intervention with her clients, she was able to change it. She was able to begin to identify when her fear of a couple's quarrel came up, and in the immediate moment she could correct her response in terms of the here-and-now reality. Thus she could learn to remind her inner self that these were not her parents, but Margaret and Dan K, to whom she had a professional responsibility.

Second, her instructor helped her to accept that the old pattern, while unhelpful in her chosen profession, only pointed out an area where she needed to learn a new behavior. It did not mean she was not a worthwhile person, nor that she could not become an effective professional helper. This again illustrates that self-acceptance must go hand in hand with self-awareness (Bate, 1968).

Influence of Other Childhood Experiences

There are other childhood experiences that, unexamined, may get in the way of effective helping. For example, if we were the child of alcoholic parents, we shall need to work at reminding ourselves in professional contacts that these alcoholic client couples are not our parents. Although their behavior toward their children triggers at times the troubled child still within us, we are safe, because this is the here and now. They are who they are and I am who I am. Thus it is my adult self who is in charge of what I think, feel, and do in this situation, not my hurt child.

Some students entering social work programs need to examine whether or not they have been able to resolve the pain they may be carrying from childhood experiences in dysfunctional families. In some instances counseling, or self-help groups, perhaps focusing on Inner Child work, may be advisable (Corey and Corey 1993: 198-199).

Expression of Feelings

The second area of self-perception identified by Cournoyer has to do with the rules in our family of origin about the expression of feelings–anger, sadness, fear, joy–and rules about how we were disciplined (1991:14, 15). These rules may have been so deeply inculcated in us while growing up that we are unaware how they automatically influence our behavior.

In some families the children's feelings are respected and accepted as real, and deserving of concerned parental attention. In others this may be true only of some feelings.

> In Karen's family she and her siblings discovered very early that crying–about anything–was unacceptable. It made their father angry. They were "crybabies" and didn't realize how lucky they were to have a good home, warm beds, good meals, and warm clothes in the winter. Their mother's response was that they must not cry because they knew it "upset Dad" and also because "nobody wants weepy kids around." They were never comforted by either parent.
>
> Karen and her three siblings learned at a very young age not to cry, unless they were alone. They also learned that "good people don't cry" and that if you cry people won't love you.
>
> Early in Karen's first practicum, at a drug abuse detox center, she saw an eighteen-year-old female client named Leanne who was about to be discharged, having completed the residential program. Her mother had refused to let her come home to live while she entered a daytime follow-up program. In telling Karen about this, Leanne started to cry bitterly. Karen's recording showed that she tried to get Leanne to stop crying, offering suggestions about not "wallowing in self-pity" and pointing out how lucky Leanne was to have a workable alternative; her aunt and uncle had offered her a home with them.

Discussion

In discussions with her field instructor, Karen made the connection between her reaction to the girl's crying and her childhood family's "rule." Karen was shocked to find that, faced with her first experience of a client's distress, she had reacted almost exactly as her own parents had. She said she had thought that her troubled childhood would be an asset to her as a social worker, as it would help her identify with how unhappy children felt. Her instructor was able to help Karen with her feelings of guilt and inadequacy.

This student learned that by identifying the source of her inappropriate response and recontacting her own childhood feelings, she could change her reaction to a client's expression of sadness by accepting their right and need to cry.

It is appropriate here to discuss the question of a student's having had prior experience as a client of social workers. For some people these experiences may be motivating factors for choosing the profession. If their experience has been a good one, they may want to make that kind of difference in others' lives (Corey and Corey, 1993:4). For some, however, the experience may not have been so happy. The motivation here may include a determination that "I'll never treat anyone the way that worker treated me!"

While this is a laudable resolve, and–sad to say–there may be justification for it, there is a danger that this student may at first be overprotective of his or her clients. Concerned about being punitive, he or she may find it very difficult to hold them to expectations or requirements that would be constructive for them. With help, however, this can be effectively resolved by the recognition of the source of the difficulty, the need for self-awareness, and recognition of the worker's responsibility in the client's reality situation.

Another kind of inappropriate use of a beginner's own experience is shown in the following:

> Catherine was a mature student, a single mother with two teenage children when she came into the MSW program. She had a BA in psychology, had married immediately after graduating, and did not work outside the home thereafter. After eight years of marriage her husband left her and moved out west. His support for her and the children was very erratic and she had worked as a legal secretary for four years after he left. Her parents were very supportive and were lending her the money to get her MSW. She felt this was more realistic than

undertaking the lengthy process of qualifying as a registered psychologist, her original career goal.

In her first practicum Catherine was working with a small group of single mothers in a public housing complex, who had been identified by the housing authority social worker as having problems with budgets, housekeeping standards, and parenting skills. Their children ranged in age from infancy to twelve years.

Catherine's recording showed clearly that she frequently made excuses for these women. She was not holding them to reasonable and agreed-upon expectations. The group meetings tended to consist of lengthy venting sessions about their struggles. Catherine never intervened to refocus on action possibilities or agreed-upon goals for change. She was the empathic, reflective listener par excellence.

Discussion

In discussing this pattern with her field instructor–the Housing Authority social worker–Catherine realized that she was very conscious of the difficult situation of these women as compared with her own. As a single mother herself she knew that even with the advantages that she had–a good education, supportive well-to-do parents a day's drive away–it still was not an easy task.

Catherine realized that she was so determined not to take the attitude that "I'm doing it and it's tough, so what's your problem?" that she was bending over backwards to "go easy" on her clients. She was overprotecting them and setting low expectations that– completely unintentionally–were in fact disrespectful and unhelpful.

Catherine's field instructor helped her to sort out these inappropriate feelings, without self-blame, and to accept that they had led her–with unquestionably good intentions–to be unhelpful.

> She changed her mode of working with the group, asking for and sometimes offering suggestions about courses of action. She was afraid that the women might reject her new approach and was agreeably surprised when at one meeting one of the women interrupted a string of complaints from another member and said, kindly but firmly, "OK, Marg, OK,

but let's look at what you can *do* about that." Later on two of the women told her after the session that they were "getting a lot more out of the meetings lately."

A significant aspect of the examples cited above is that in each case the instructor helped students not to judge themselves harshly for the practice errors that were identified. Students needed to accept that the unhelpful intervention was simply an indication of who they were at that point in time and what they needed to learn from the experience. It did not make them persons of lesser value, nor did it mean that they could not become effective helpers.

In summary, then, the worker's acceptance of self, of strengths, limitations, and areas of difficulty, without self-blame, is an important first step in the development of professional helping skills. Accepting ourselves as we are frees us to make changes as we find them appropriate and necessary. We can incorporate new information to make constructive changes in thinking, feeling, and acting. This is how we grow and develop toward our full potential as persons and professional helpers.

Only when we fully accept ourselves as we are, can we genuinely accept our clients as they truly are. Biestek states that "Self-awareness leads to the acceptance of self and ultimately to the acceptance of others" (1957:80).

THE WORKER'S NEEDS

The third area of the "self as instrument" that we need to examine is that of our own needs. We all bring various needs into our work situation, and in social work, Corey and Corey point out that our own needs can work either for or against our being truly helpful to our clients (1993:3). It is not a question of our needs being—of themselves—an obstacle to effective help, only that we must examine whether we are meeting those needs appropriately or inappropriately in our practice (1993:8).

Corey and Corey's chapter on needs and motivation is valuable reading for students (1993:1-29). They list an extensive number of needs they see as requiring attention to ensure that they do not hinder our work with clients. We need to develop self-awareness about our needs and how they can affect us in the helping relationship role. The six needs identified below are selected from an earlier work of the same authors with some amendments from their current edition. These appear to me to be representative and useful here.

- the need for control and power;
- the need to be nurturing;
- the need to change others in the direction of our own values;
- the need to provide answers;
- the need for feeling adequate, particularly when it becomes overly important that the client confirm our competence; and
- the need to be respected and appreciated. (Corey and Corey, 1990:62)

In looking at this list we can recognize that control, nurturing, and focus on change are constructive in professional helping. We shall not be helpful if we do not maintain some control of the process. Some of our clients do require a strong nurturing component in the relationship because they never had anyone who really cared about their struggles. Change is the prime objective of social work service. Are these not healthy needs for the social worker?

The critical factor here is the focus of need-meeting. The question we must ask ourselves is, whose needs are being met?

Control and power are qualities that are particularly vulnerable to abuse, in professional helping as in other relationships. We need to remember, as stated earlier, that while power is more integral to some professional roles–probation and child protection, for example–than others, there is some element of power in most social work positions. As noted earlier, we need to distinguish between authority and power, and to be watchful that we do not abuse either in our practice.

We may find ourselves overexerting control in our professional relationships and we need to look at where this need comes from. Is it to relieve some inner anxiety of our own? Is it to reassure us of our own adequacy as persons? When we examine how and in precisely what circumstances we are exercising control with our clients, we can determine if we are exercising it for the sake of our own need to control, or if it is truly in the clients' interests in their individual situation.

Corey and Corey suggest we ask ourselves what is our purpose in helping; is it "to control the lives of others, or to teach them to regain effective control of their own lives?" (1993:8).

Our need to be nurturing can degenerate into an automatic response that does not carefully assess the needs of this client or group of clients. As stated earlier, some of our clients are literally starved for a caring relationship and it is appropriate that we offer them this quality in our counseling. However, we need to remember always that the objective of such nurture is the fostering of personal growth. It is disrespectful and unhelpful for us to infantilize our clients by over-protection, too much "doing for" and so on. This may stem from some aspect of our own need to nurture.

Early in my own practice (I was in my mid-thirties and my children in their early teens), I was seeing for the second time in her own home a twenty-year-old woman whose husband had left her for another woman when their second baby was a few weeks old. Although the relationship had been stormy ever since the marriage, Debbie was heartbroken and terrified for her own and her children's future. On my first visit we had talked about social assistance for single mothers; she was receiving emergency social assistance while that was being processed.

They had married—against their parents' wishes—because of Debbie's pregnancy. Debbie had never felt her parents (especially her mother) really cared about her. In the present emergency they were totally unsympathetic, taking the attitude that she had chosen to go against their wishes and must suffer the consequences. Larry's parents had never acknowledged her or the children.

Talking about this, Debbie, sitting at the other end of the couch from me, began to cry bitterly. She was a slight woman with long blonde hair. She looked very young and vulnerable and it hurt me to see her so alone and deeply hurt. I moved over to her and took her in my arms. I felt her accept my comfort for a couple of moments, but she very quickly got up, went to get some tissues, and stopped crying.

She did not return to her seat, and for the rest of the interview remained standing behind the couch where I was still sitting. This clearly told me: "Keep your distance!" I realized that I had intruded on her in a disrespectful way. Perhaps it was even more important that in doing so I had blocked her need to let go and cry.

Discussion

Talking this over with my supervisor, I realized that in acting as I did, it was *my* distress for her that I was trying to relieve. I was meeting my own need, not hers. I was reminded of my MSW field instructor's injunction "Don't do, just be!" It was hard for me simply to be with her in her pain, yet that was what she needed. Debbie taught me a valuable lesson about when and how to offer physical comfort.

The need to change others in the direction of our own values is linked to the need to provide ready answers to people's problems. Like the other needs identified here, these do not necessarily reflect unethical motivations, but despite good intentions, without adequate self-awareness, such modes of response can get in the way of our practice (Corey and Corey, 1993:7). Our answers may simply not fit this person or group of persons. We must pay careful attention to the individuality of each client or group of clients or we shall severely limit their self-determination. This can block them from actively involving themselves in the helping process.

The need to feel adequate is a common trouble spot, particularly, as Corey and Corey say, as it often becomes overly important for us that the clients confirm our competence (1993:6). We can be tripped up here when clients—for example, in an action-oriented group—decide to undertake a course of action that is different from that which we have believed and suggested was the productive one. In their rejection of what we believe is the "right" way to solve their problem, we may feel as if they have rejected us. We may also feel inadequate if their course of action proves them right.

In these experiences we need to examine just how our own need to "be right" and to be "successful" denies the clients their right to self-determination. We shall correct this through the practice of self-awareness and careful attention to accepting that we can be "wrong" and still be worthwhile persons and useful helpers.

Sometimes we can be overcome with feelings of inadequacy and failure when our clients do not adequately resolve the difficulties that brought them to us. This may threaten our need for professional "success," and our need for clients to demonstrate growth in self-reliance and in coping with their lives. Corey and Corey state that

> If you depend exclusively on your clients to feel like a useful human being, your self-worth is on shaky ground. (1993:6)

We must learn to let go of the idea that we can help everyone and accept that we simply do not "click" with some people. Some are not ready to make the kinds of changes that would lead to greater happiness and well-being, and there will always be some whom we cannot help find "the key" that could move them out of self-defeating patterns. This does not mean we are incompetent. It is simply a realistic acceptance of ourselves as professional helpers with limitations as well as strengths.

In conclusion, Lammert states that

> Being aware of one's moment-to-moment experience, cognitively sorting it out, and processing it in terms of what we know about ourselves and our clients enables us to move quickly and gracefully between feeling "with" or joining the client and having a solid sense of our own separateness. This process is *a part of good therapeutic work.* (1986:376, emphasis added)

SUMMARY OF MAIN POINTS

1. Self-awareness is a key principle in professional social work. It has been identified as being a critical factor that distinguishes the effective helper.
2. Without self-awareness we may distort what our clients express or how we respond—sometimes both—by inappropriate reactions.

3. The student initially needs to look into him or herself and seek to answer the question "Who am I as a thinking, feeling, relating, and acting person?" This can be examined under three headings:

   • beliefs, opinions, and values
   • self-perception, and
   • needs

4. Our beliefs, opinions, and values commonly include biases and prejudices that can get in the way of our being truly helpful.
5. Our self-perception is a function of our family of origin, our relationships with others, and how we have dealt with experience up to this point in our lives. It comprises our level of self-esteem, the expectations we have of others, and our way of responding to them.
6. Familial experiences from an early age can influence us by assigning us—or by our assigning ourselves—one or more roles as a family member.
7. Family rules may have conditioned us concerning the expression of certain feelings. Unexamined, these automatic responses can seriously interfere with our effectiveness in helping.
8. We need to become aware of our own needs, as persons and professional helpers, and to ensure that in a given intervention we are meeting the clients' needs and not our own. Second, we must guard against requiring our clients to meet our needs.
9. Self-awareness needs to be a constant, moment-to-moment habit in all our professional contacts.

REFERENCES

Bate, Clive C. (1968). "Mistake-Making, Congruency and Self-Acceptance as Helping Tools." *The Social Worker*, 36(2):2-98.

Biestek, Felix P. (1957). *The Casework Relationship*. Chicago, IL: Loyola University Press.

Combs, Arthur W., Donald Avila, and William Purkey. (1973). *Helping Relationships: Basic Concepts for the Helping Professions*. Boston: Allyn and Bacon, Inc.

Corey, Marianne Schneider and Gerald Corey. (1990). *Becoming a Helper, First Edition*. Pacific Grove, CA: Brooks/Cole Publishing Co., p. 62.

——— (1993). *Becoming a Helper, Second Edition*. Pacific Grove, CA: Brooks/Cole Publishing Co., Chapter 1.

Cournoyer, Barry. (1991). *Social Work Skills Workbook*. Belmont, CA: Wadsworth Publishing, pp. 10-42.

Lammert, Marilyn. (1986). "Experience as Knowing: Utilizing Therapist Self-Awareness." *Social Casework: The Journal of Contemporary Social Work*, 67(6):369-376.

Chapter 6

Acceptance:
Creating the Climate for Change

Acceptance of persons as they are, however they present themselves to us and for whatever reasons, is a critical element in the helping relationship; indeed, without it we cannot help people. Our help is effective to the degree that we accept each client the way he or she is: that we are not shocked, frightened, or overwhelmed by their ideas, feelings, or behavior. This is a specific practice application of our respect for human worth and dignity, and is a quality that we need to cultivate in ourselves as a professional practice principle.

Biestek defines acceptance as:

> an action principle wherein the [worker] perceives and deals with each client as he/she really is, including [their] strengths and weaknesses, congenial and uncongenial qualities, [their] positive and negative feelings, constructive and destructive attitudes and behaviour, maintaining consistently a sense of the client's innate dignity and personal worth. (1957:72)

It is important that we understand that we are required to accept each client not in spite of, but with all the aspects noted above–the uncongenial qualities and/or destructive, antisocial behavior that in many instances are a large part of the reason they need our help. The foulmouthed sullenness of the delinquent teenager; the outrage of the physically abusive father who asserts that his own childhood beatings "made a man of me!"; the elaborate psychospiritual phraseology of the well-educated adult child of alcoholic parents that obstructs down-to-earth discussion–all such qualities can "put us off" initially. Biestek says that

> the extremely vital point is that the [social] worker, while seeing the client's negatives realistically, maintains an equally real respect for him. (1957:71)

At first contact we need to accept that these are part of how this person is coping with the experience of asking for, or being told that they need, our help. We do not know at this point to what degree these may be habitual defenses used in coping with other life events.

THE OBJECT OF ACCEPTANCE

Siporin states that

> The application of the principle of acceptance results in the lowering of the client's anxieties, an increase in his/her self-respect and self-esteem, the facilitation of client expression of feelings, [and] the building of trust between the worker and the client. . . . (1975:76)

Clients can feel safe in letting down some of their habitual defenses when they feel respected and accepted, in the fullest sense, as who they are, by someone who is empathically trying to understand how this experience feels to them. They can then begin to look at their difficulty in a more realistic way (Biestek, 1957:72).

This is the object of acceptance–to free the client to feel safe in being him or herself, as the starting point for examining the possibility and the potential value of change. Combs, Avila, and Purkey state succinctly that

> Growth cannot proceed from where people are not, it can only proceed from where people are. (1973:228)

Acceptance must always include the expectation that every human being has the potential for growth and change. This may present some difficulty in certain instances. In corrections, we may face it early on in working with persons whose criminal—perhaps repulsive—behavior appears to be a well-established habit of living. In other cases, after some purposeful work with little change in attitudes, feelings, or behavior, we may want to "give up" on the person, rather than accepting that they are not ready to move at our planned pace toward constructive change. We need to remember that the objective of acceptance is therapeutic, in that it creates the climate that can foster that growth and change (Biestek, 1957:71; Rogers, 1980:115).

The therapeutic purpose of acceptance as a key to helping people effect change in their lives also requires us to make the distinction between "acceptance" and "approval." We have to learn to accept the person—for example, the man who has sexually abused his nine-year-old stepdaughter for the past two years, and her mother who told her to "stop making up filthy stories." But in accepting them as persons who have behaved in this way, we are not joining them in minimizing the injury done to this little girl. Biestek defines the therapeutic focus of acceptance as "pertinent reality" (1957:72). The pertinent reality in such a case is that the behavior of both these parents was unacceptable. In our culture the stepfather's actions were criminal and the mother's behavior was morally and legally a breach of our society's family values in denying the child the protection she was entitled to expect from her caregivers. This is the pertinent reality with which we must help these persons deal.

THE PERSON IS NOT THE BEHAVIOR

As noted earlier, in holding on to our principle of accepting the person, while not approving of what they have done, we need to differentiate between the core identity of the person and that person's behavior. In North American culture this is not an easy task. In general, many of our clients have grown up with parent figures who have identified behavior with the person. In many families disobedience, displaying a bad temper, or lying are seen, from an early age, not as a child's mistaken experiments in learning how to survive and cope with adult, sociocultural expectations, but as the behavior of a "Bad Child." Rogers says that repeated expressions of parental disapproval of "the child's spontaneous feelings and real attitudes [lead to the child's belief that he or she is] a person whom no one could love" (1980:226).

This label becomes part of that child's self-perception as he or she grows. Outside the family, society also tends to label persons based on their behavior, which later confirms the adult child in his or her self-evaluation. Thus it is often very difficult for our clients to recognize and accept that the kind of judgments we make are of their behavior and not of them as persons.

This distinction between behavior and personal identity is, in my own experience, a difficult obstacle to overcome for many workers. The cultural labelling noted above can affect anyone's reaction to criticism. Some students react to a poor grade on an assignment or critical comments on a midterm evaluation as a criticism of them as persons and of their potential for professional practice.

I have found it helpful to explain to students and clients that what we are examining and evaluating is simply whether or not a specific item of their behavior effectively serves the purpose for which it is designed. The rating has relevance only insofar as it indicates a need for useful change–for students seeking to realize career objectives or for clients seeking to improve their social functioning.

I learned something about the difference between labelling the person and identifying the behavior from one of my clients early in my practice in a child welfare setting.

> Because I knew that AA defines an alcoholic as anyone whose drinking causes problems in their life, I said to a client once, "I believe you're an alcoholic, Mr. G." He raised his voice and said I didn't know what I was talking about, he wasn't going to be insulted in his own home, etc., etc. I said, "Just a minute, Mr. G. I didn't say your were a 'lush'; I didn't say you were a 'lousy drunk.' I believe that when you start to drink you can't stop, and that's creating a lot of problems for you here at home. That's what AA calls an 'alcoholic.' " He calmed down somewhat and we discussed the problems that his most recent binge had created: neighbors had called the police and our agency–not for the first time–because of the ensuing uproar between him and his wife.

CREATING THE CLIMATE FOR CHANGE

Rogers lists three basic attributes of the effective helper in creating a climate for change. These are genuineness (which he clarifies as realness or congruence), unconditional positive regard, and empathic understanding. He equates unconditional positive regard with acceptance and sees it as our key to empathic understanding (1980:115-117). This level of understanding makes it possible for us to enter into each client's reality, not simply at the feeling level, but with a therapeutic focus.

Biestek identifies three steps to the action of acceptance:

(i) perceiving: we must see objectively what we are accepting;
(ii) therapeutic understanding: we must see the interrelationship of the presenting problem; the situation of needing help, what each of these means to this person, and how it all relates to the helping process of therapeutic change; and
(iii) acknowledging the totality of the person: their past and present actions, perceptions, and feelings as a pertinent reality. (1957:70)

This concept of "pertinent reality" is echoed by Goldstein, who reminds us that "reality is not an objective fact" (1983:268). He adds that

> What we believe our world to be like justifies our actions in that world; the perceived consequences of actions are used to verify beliefs. (1983:271)

Goldstein's reminder is important as we consciously undertake Biestek's three steps in acceptance. We must perceive clearly, understand, and accept that this highly individualized perception of reality colors each situation or set of circumstances that each client or group of clients brings to us for help to make constructive changes. This is real for them, whether they come to us voluntarily or under some external mandate. As discussed earlier, they have very specific anxieties about this situation, and particularly about whether they will be accepted as who they really are.

The Client's Anxieties

Earlier we examined some of the feelings and needs of the person who comes to us for professional help. We need to perceive objectively what part these needs play in the way this person (or persons) present at the first contact. As noted above, we need to be cautious about identifying behavior we observe at this point as being part of the client's overall problem. It may simply be his or her response to the immediate situation of asking for help or being told they must receive it.

First then, there is the anxiety about what kind of person we are. Are we going to judge and condemn? Are we going to be shocked—as some of their friends or relatives have been—if they express negative feelings about events or people in their lives? Biestek points out that the client may even be protecting him or herself from some of these negative feelings, terrified that these make him or her a "bad person" (1957:76), perhaps even unacceptable as a member of the human family. Biestek states that it is vitally important that we create an atmosphere of safety by our acceptance, such that "the need to protect himself [from these feelings] can be lessened" (1957:76).

Second, is this professional person's accepting attitude genuine? Biestek says that our acceptance needs to be genuine and continuous throughout every aspect of our intervention. It needs to become truly a part of our self-as-instrument. Biestek states that this quality contains both thought and feeling elements, of which the thought component includes our awareness of therapeutic purpose and our knowledge of human personality and behavior (1957:78-79). In this connection Goldstein cites Laing's warning about the "screen of theory," in that we need to be careful that our theoretical knowledge does not "further separate [us] from the client's actual world of experience" (1983:271). Goldstein further states that

> "How is it for you in your terms?" endows the embryonic relationship with qualities of mutuality and respect and affirms the client's authority about his or her own values, motives and way of life. (1983:271)

This approach safeguards against the premature categorization of persons and/or behavior. Having decided that diagnostically two and two make four, the danger is that we then develop a need to minimize—even ignore—the entrance of a new factor that changes the equation. Our cognitive reaction to troubled persons must be as continually dynamic and open to new information as is our feeling response.

Third, we also know that clients bring to the helping process a dual attitude—what Goldstein calls "the will to change tempered by a resistance to grow or to accept help" (1983:267). This ambivalence about the risks and potential value of change is a universal human characteristic—to which we ourselves are not immune—and we must accept that it may permeate at least the early stages of the helping process. If clients experience some rewards from new behavior, the ambivalence may be reduced.

Fourth, Goldstein reminds us that there are "no familiar guidelines or clues" for clients in this situation at first encounter. Even what is being offered to them—just what is "counseling?"—may initially seem not at all clear, leaving clients with the feeling of being "at sea." There may also be cultural barriers for many clients, perhaps against discussing personal problems with anyone "outside the family." Even the words we use may carry a different meaning to individual clients, depending on their idiosyncratic or culturally influenced perceptions of our role in their lives (1983:268-269).

The Worker's Role

The clients' anxieties noted above may reflect beliefs, feelings, and attitudes about life in general. Our full acceptance of the total person, and our willingness to learn and understand their total reality is the first factor in creating the climate for change.

The second factor is our readiness and ability to help clients begin to express their beliefs, feelings, and attitudes toward the trouble that brings them to us. We need to accept that this may, in come cases, be a very different perception of their life situation from the way it appears to us. Our acceptance of this as being their reality is the beginning of what Rogers has called "empathic understanding" (1980:116).

Biestek states that our acceptance here must be genuinely based in each client's individual readiness and apparent capacity for making changes (1957:79). There is a danger that in applying a belief in client potential for growth and change, in general, without individualized attention, we may give some clients the feeling that we cannot accept their reluctance, or their uncertainty about the advantages for them in such change. We may subtly load them with a "should" that implies we do not accept who and where they are at this time. We need to remember that our concern is "not the good, but the real" (Biestek, 1957:72). Thus our professional responsibility is to create the climate in which this person or group of persons feels safe in beginning to examine the need for change at their own pace, and in the manner that is workable for them.

Nicole M. came to the Family Counseling Center asking for advice about her relationship with her husband. In making the appointment on the phone, she said he had refused to consider counseling for both of them. He said the problems were entirely hers, and she felt he was right. Gail, the Intake worker, agreed to see her alone to talk about what marriage counseling involved, and suggested that perhaps with such information, and the agency's leaflet, Nicole could convince her husband to come with her.

Nicole, aged thirty-one, a full-time homemaker with three children–three, four, and seven years old–described feeling that she "does so many things the wrong way" and that this aggravates her husband, Larry. This situation started about four years ago, and has become increasingly difficult for her. Nicole became teary-eyed about the "rotten names" Larry frequently calls her–almost daily. She believes that most of it is "her fault" because she is not well-organized and finds it hard to be "always thinking about how he likes things to be done" when she is pressed for time. He often becomes very angry when she does not want sex because of how she feels about the way he talks to her. Whenever she refuses him he reminds her about her marriage vows, and then she feels very guilty.

Her husband is in business for himself. He lost a considerable amount of money almost three years ago in breaking up a disastrous partnership. Since he went on his own things have greatly improved financially. He is now doing quite well and is very well thought of in the community. They have a very busy social life, involving a lot of entertaining of business associates in their own home. They are invited out a lot, and attend various community events because Larry says they "must keep in the mainstream" for the sake of his business. Larry wants her to be more involved in community life–committees or volunteer work–and he feels she "ought to support his career more" in these ways. She finds the house, the children, and the entertaining keep her very busy. If she were better organized, she says, she would be able to do what he wants. She feels badly that she cannot support him in this way, "like the other wives" in their circle.

Nicole said she has help in the house one half day every two weeks (Larry says that is all they can afford while they are recovering from the losses of the earlier business failure). She has stopped asking him for more help because it "makes him very angry." He says he cannot afford to "subsidize my incompetence." She has no idea what the family's income is or how their past debts now stand.

He gets very angry if things are not the way he likes them– dinner being late, the children's table manners, the arrangement of his incoming mail on his desk at home according to the size of the envelopes, etc.

Gail asked how Larry expressed his anger. Nicole replied that he "shouts and calls her awful names." She shrugged and said occasionally he "pushes me about." When asked to explain, Nicole very hesitantly said he sometimes hits her about the face and shoulders "a bit." Yes, sometimes she has bruises, but "no broken bones or anything serious like that." She half-laughed and said Gail must not get the idea that she was a "battered wife." Larry does not drink and he has a college degree in Business Administration. He only hits her "when she has disappointed or aggravated him."

Larry has said he does not need counseling, but he believes Nicole does, because he feels she has a "mental problem." For a while she thought he was right, but lately she thinks the problem is just her inability to organize her time. She feels she needs counseling to help her to be better organized and take more control of her home and social obligations.

Gail, a committed feminist, recognizing the typical pattern of the battered wife, suggested that Nicole talk to an agency staff member who specialized in counseling "abused women." Nicole reacted strongly against this, repeating that she was not a "battered wife." She reiterated the distinction she had made earlier of their solid, well-educated, professional background as–in her mind–proof of this. Larry would not get so angry if she were a "better wife and homemaker."

In response to Gail's statement that no woman "deserves to be physically attacked," Nicole said she felt that some men were more hot-tempered than others and that Larry had a "short fuse." She asked if there was anyone on the staff who specialized in time management and domestic organization problems. Gail replied that this could be arranged but that she believed that Nicole needed to look at her situation with less self-blame and more concern for her own well-being.

She offered Nicole an appointment with a therapist who worked with women who were being abused. Nicole thanked her and said she would call if she decided to follow through. Two months later Nicole still had not contacted the agency about an appointment.

Discussion

This example illustrates the point noted above: the need to accept not only the client's view of the problem, but also the pace at which this person is able to address it. For most workers, committed feminists or not, Nicole's presentation would immediately arouse concern and perhaps some anger–certainly at Larry, perhaps at her–at the way in which he has convinced Nicole of his "diagnosis" of their problems. But this is the pertinent reality of the situation for Nicole. There is one tiny crack in her acceptance of Larry's overall "rightness"–she disagrees that she has a "mental problem." This could have been reenforced and used had counseling been offered at a level that Nicole was ready to accept.

Undoubtedly Gail genuinely empathized with this woman's distress, and certainly her concern was valid, but she could not accept that this client was clearly not able, at that point, to look at herself as an abused wife, or at Larry as an abusive husband. Pushing a program that directly addressed the abuse convinced this client that the worker did not understand her struggle. To reiterate the statement quoted earlier, Nicole could not grow from where Gail perceived her as being, she could only grow from where she was, and at her own pace.[1]

It has been noted above that our active acceptance must include both thought and feeling elements (Biestek, 1957:79). The cognitive element requires first the recognition of our therapeutic purpose in helping, and second, the appropriate use of our knowledge of human behavior in the social environment. But the purposeful application of knowledge will not be helpful–it may even be harmful–without what many writers have called "the disciplined use of self," the essential tool of practice.

This use of self is, as described earlier, key to constructive helping in social work, and the essential principle here is our responsibility for self-awareness. We need to accept ourselves with the same compassionate recognition of what is real for us that we use in accepting what is real for our clients. This acceptance of self allows us–as it does our clients–to let down our defenses; it allows us to admit mistakes and try to correct them with our clients. Empathic understanding in the relationship involves our caring as deeply and genuinely as possible about each person who needs our professional help while maintaining a level of objectivity about their life situation and the changes that they need to make. This facilitates our shared objective of their becoming more comfortable in all their relationships, happier, stronger, more productive, and more confident that "it is safe–okay–to be *me*."

OBSTACLES TO ACCEPTANCE

The inability to accept the client's level of readiness to work on the presenting problem can, as we have seen, get in the way of our acceptance of each person or group of persons and thus block our helpfulness. Biestek is reassuring that we cannot expect to acquire perfect acceptance, and that our level of capacity to accept our clients can vary "from day to day or from client to client" (1957: 81). What is important is that we recognize our need for improvement and that we strive continually toward greater skill in the acceptance of the people we serve. Biestek lists several obstacles to our acceptance (1957:81-87), some of which have been mentioned above; others will now be discussed.

Insufficient Knowledge of Human Behavior

The more we know about patterns of human behavior–about the common emotional reactions to interpersonal relationships and to life events, whether perceived as stressful or "normal"–the better we are able to comprehend struggles that our clients experience. We need to have a good grasp of the defense mechanisms frequently employed by human beings in our culture. We need also to learn about the sociocultural forces that affect the responses of persons nurtured in a culture other than our own. In sum, a broad base of psychosocial knowledge is vital in enabling us to accept fully who our clients are, and the nature of their trouble; why they perceive their situation in a particular way and how their response to it helps or hinders them from resolving the issues effectively.

Nonacceptance of Something in Self

Unresolved issues in ourselves can seriously get in the way of our objectivity in assessing and helping clients to act upon a particular difficulty. This can make us anxious, and block our acceptance of the client's difficulty. Then we may not be able to help them face and begin to deal with it realistically.

> Darren, a worker in family service, had never fully faced and let go of his anger against his father, who deserted the family when Darren, aged eleven, was the eldest of four siblings. His mother and uncle had told him he was "the man of the family now." He became very anxious when Alan, his twenty-year-old client, said "My father wants us to get to know each other now that I am working and away from home, but sometimes I still really hate him for leaving us the way he did." Darren felt very anxious and disapproving. He asked, "How does your mother feel about you seeing your father?" Alan replied, "I know I shouldn't feel that way, I feel bad

about hating my father." Darren repeated the question about Alan's mother.

Discussion

Alan's response was an immediate clue to his feeling of being rejected by Darren. A worker more comfortable with his own feelings could have picked that up and have admitted that his changing the subject was not appropriate. This could have helped Alan in beginning to express his anger, but Darren's unresolved feelings and his lack of self-awareness blocked his ability to accept this client's negative feelings and thus prevented him from being helpful.

No one can tell another person how they "should" feel. The constructive response to such expressions is an explicit acceptance that that is how they *do* feel. This can lead to exploring the reasons for such feelings and the merits of letting them go. Biestek points out that while we are not happy that our client has such negative feelings, we can be happy that he or she has felt safe to express them. In this way a real and very relevant part of the client's struggle is out in the open where it can be addressed as part of their pertinent reality (1957:77).

Imputing One's Own Feelings to the Client

The emphasis here is again on the need for self-awareness. We have all heard from family or friends, "If I were in your shoes I would do this or that. . . ." Our inner feeling, whether we express it or not, is: "Maybe so, but *I'm* in my shoes, not you," and we feel that what our difficulty means to us has not been heard. The perception, significance, and meaning of any experience, struggle, or choice with which a person is faced are, in their entirety, highly individual. While some aspects of a response may be shared in common with others, the totality of the struggle's meaning is specific to each individual. Suggesting "I think I would feel (this way or that)" denies this. Biestek says that

> dealing with the client as if [he or she] were someone else is experienced by the client as subtle rejection. (1957:82-83)

Biases and Prejudices

As discussed in a previous chapter, early in our professional education we begin to strive for self-awareness in the more common types of prejudice—race, religion, economic status, etc. There are, however, more subtle kinds of bias and prejudice that can be obstacles to our full acceptance of the pertinent reality of some of our clients. Some of these may arise from a confirmed but unexamined opinion about the cause of certain difficulties or the best solution. For example, a "conviction that adoption is the best plan for all children born to [single] mothers can prevent the worker . . . from dealing with the full reality" of certain cases (Biestek, 1957:83).

Such obstacles to our full acceptance can also come about because of our overenthusiastic commitment to certain theories of human behavior or even to certain intervention models (Goldstein, 1983:270). As noted above, we must continually be on guard to submit our theory base to careful, objective examination, and we must be open to integrating new information into a meaningful analysis of what this individual's behavior means in his or her life situation.

Unwarranted Reassurances

Reassurance can be an important factor in support of a client as long as it is based on a realistic view of the situation being discussed. If our reassurance is not based on reality but on what we think or wish reality to be, it comes across as rejection—of the client's feelings about the problem, their anxiety, their reluctance about making a decision or of taking some action, or their fear of its consequences (Biestek, 1957:83).

Adult clients who are returning to school to upgrade their employment skills need us to accept that they are really scared about the undertaking. If we say "Of course you'll pass this course with flying colors!" we are not accepting their feelings. We may or may not be genuine in our assertion. We may be feeling uncertain ourselves about the plan and its outcome and perhaps feel we dare not suggest that the client's plan is unrealistic at this time. Either way, the clients will feel that we do not accept where they are and do not understand their feelings.

The realistic way of approaching such a situation is to accept the feelings of anxiety as real, and to reexamine the factors, pro and con, that went into the decision to go back to school.

Loss of Respect for the Client

So many of our clients, as has been said, come to us with damaged self-esteem. Some have never developed a basic sense of self-worth. Others have lost a perhaps fragile self-esteem because of repeated experiences that they and/or their interpersonal world have categorized as failures. They need our reassurance that in spite of this, they are entitled to our respect because of their innate human worth and dignity as unique individuals. Biestek warns that our acceptance of clients can be gravely damaged if we begin to lose respect for them (1957:85-86).

Dwayne, aged twenty-two, was admitted to the hospital after making a suicide gesture, following a six-month history of being fired from various jobs. Having trained as an auto mechanic, he graduated from community college and moved out west to a large city where he believed there were "lots of jobs." He had heard this from a friend, but made no preliminary inquiries. Having grown up in a small city, he felt insecure in the big city atmosphere, did not know where to begin, and became too anxious to hunt for a job effectively.

He came back to live at home, applied for social assistance, and started looking for work there. Things were slow in his hometown, unemployment was running higher than usual, but he got a job with an acquaintance of his father's.

This lasted for two months. Dwayne was fired because he complained that he was not getting the kind of work experience that would advance his career and help him to get his certification papers. At the insistence of his father he took another job almost immediately, one offered by a friend of his brother-in-law. This was only part-time. Dwayne became very dissatisfied with the arrangement and complained that others were being given the chance to work more hours than he was. His boss there told him that part of the problem was that some of the employees would not work with him because of his "attitude" and that he would do well to "smarten up."

Dwayne took great exception to this, and quit. Two or three more work experiences of similar short duration followed, ending either in his quitting or being fired. During this time he was seeing a girlfriend and talked of marriage. She was a receptionist in a business office, and told him there was no question of their marrying until he was working steadily. The loss of two more jobs provoked her to end the relationship.

Dwayne stayed at home for about two weeks, staying in bed (or up, but in pajamas and housecoat), watching TV. When his father told him to either start looking for work or leave home, Dwayne cut the back of his wrists severely with a razor blade and was admitted to hospital.

Karl, an experienced psychiatric social worker, saw Dwayne while he was in hospital, and continued to work with him in out-patient after-care. He also saw his parents. Karl could see that while Dwayne's parents had given him financial security and met his material needs more than adequately, it seemed there had been little real affection or caring concern in the home. Some of Dwayne's ways of expressing his feelings (especially his anger "at the world") were typical of an emotionally deprived adolescent. Karl understood this, but found himself dreading his interviews with Dwayne.

He found that Dwayne consistently blamed others–his parents, his former employers and colleagues at work, his ex-girlfriend–for all his difficulties. He could not accept any responsibility for any part of his problems. Karl began to find it harder and harder to be patient listening to what he came to feel were D's "Poor Me!" stories.

Finally, after consultation with his supervisor, it was agreed that Dwayne would be assigned to another worker.

Discussion

This case illustrates how the worker's loss of respect for the client's basic worth blocked his ability to accept this individual's perception of his reality. The irritation that Karl felt blocked his objective assessment of what Dwayne was really struggling with and thus prevented his beginning constructive, therapeutic work. This worker was alert and self-aware enough to recognize that he had lost respect for his client; he had enough self-acceptance and self-confidence to face the nature of his difficulty and to share it with his supervisor. With the problem out in the open, the client's needs could be appropriately assessed and met through a change of worker. As Biestek says, our ability to respect and accept clients may vary at times. Sometimes the kind of difficulty faced by Karl in this case can be resolved in consultation with a supervisor or with peers, but if it cannot, the responsible way to handle it is by a change of worker. Where this cannot be arranged, a referral to another source of help is appropriate.

Overidentification

Overidentification occurs when we lose professional objectivity and our own feelings become involved so that we feel as if the client's troubles are actually our own. It is one aspect of our not maintaining controlled emotional involvement, which will be discussed in detail in a later chapter.

This again highlights the need for self-awareness. The clients' problems may trigger something in our own experience–an old pain that we thought was resolved, or perhaps a current, distressful life situation. Without concerned attention to self-awareness, it is possible for us to start "feeling like" our client, unconsciously feeling that the hurt or injustice has been done to us (Biestek, 1957:86).

In clinical work this may take the form of joining the adult children of alcoholics in their anger against their parents for the lack of caring and frequent broken promises. This immediately results in our losing the ability to help clients look objectively at that anger, accepting its justifiable roots, but helping them to examine what holding on to it is doing to them at the present time.

In advocacy work with community groups, our anger will render both our empowerment methods and our advocacy much less effective because it may lead us to support methods of approach that further antagonize the powers-that-be, putting them on the defensive. Our job here is to accept our clients' anger and the reality of the injustice as they see and feel it, but to help them work toward a calm marshalling of facts and figures or other resources which may be more likely to achieve the desired ends.

It is important that we accept our right to feel angry or hurt for many of our clients, both individuals and groups who have suffered or are suffering deprivation and/or injustice. I hope we never lose the capacity to feel this. However, if we are to maintain the level of professional objectivity that our clients need from us, we must recognize and deal with our anger in a way that prevents it from spilling over and complicating—even defeating—our helping efforts.

Acceptance provides the basis of the helping relationship; it enables clients to feel safe in being themselves, and safe in expressing their real thoughts and feelings "without thought of what the worker would want to hear" (Biestek, 1957:87). It is one of the essential professional principles that we must strive to achieve as a personal value and implement as a necessary aspect of helping.

SUMMARY OF MAIN POINTS

1. Our capacity for acceptance is an integral part of our disciplined, professional use of self. It involves concerned attention to self-awareness.
2. Professional responsibility demands that we strive to accept each client or group of clients as persons of innate worth and dignity with, not in spite of, their uncongenial characteristics and/or antisocial behavior.
3. The purpose of acceptance is therapeutic; it facilitates our exploration and empathic understanding of each client's pertinent reality. This last comprises the totality of their thoughts and feelings about their situation, as well as their behavioral responses to that situation.
4. We must make a clear distinction between acceptance of the person(s) and approval of their behavior.
5. Acceptance is comprised of cognitive and feeling elements, and both elements must be kept in balance, having regard always to the therapeutic purpose.
6. Acceptance includes the belief in and expectation of people's ability to grow and change, but we need to accept each person

or group's readiness for change, and the pace of working that feels comfortable for them.

7. We need be watchful of attributes, biases, or unresolved feelings of our own that create obstacles to our acceptance of our clients.

8. Overidentification with the clients' feelings can obstruct our empathic understanding, and can interfere with the implementation of what can be constructive, individualized methods of help in resolving their difficulties.

NOTE

1. It is beyond the scope of this chapter to elaborate on ethical and service-policy issues that the handling of this case may raise for discussion with students who have had work experience. (To cite one or two examples: How does the agency determine whether or not it is within family service policy to see a wife alone in such a case without her husband's involvement? How do we ensure that he knows she is receiving service and understands that the content will not be shared with him without her consent?)

REFERENCES

Biestek, Felix P. (1957). *The Casework Relationship.* Chicago, IL: Loyola University Press.

Combs, Arthur W., Donald L. Avila, and William W. Purkey. (1973). *Helping Relationships: Basic Concepts for the Helping Professions.* Boston: Allyn and Bacon, Inc.

Goldstein, Howard. (1983). "Starting Where the Client Is." *Social Casework,* 64(5):267-275.

Laing, Ronald D. (1965). *The Divided Self.* New York: Penguin.

Rogers, Carl R. (1980). *A Way of Being.* Boston: Houghton Mifflin Company.

Siporin, Max. (1975). *Introduction to Social Work Practice.* New York: Macmillan Publishing Company.

Chapter 7

The Nonjudgmental Attitude: Understanding and Evaluating, Not Assigning Blame

Social workers need to adopt the nonjudgmental attitude as a value principle so that its practice becomes part of the self-as-instrument. It is integral to the helping relationship. It may be defined as

> a quality of the helping relationship that is based on a conviction that the function of social work is not judging or assigning guilt or blame to persons, but understanding and evaluating the clients' difficulties with the objective of helping to resolve or ameliorate their problems. This understanding includes the evaluation of the clients' beliefs, attitudes, and actions, and assessing how these contribute to or inhibit their psychosocial functioning and well-being. (adapted from Biestek, 1957:90-99)

Biestek adds that "the attitude includes thought and feeling elements and is transmitted to the client" (1957:96), and further states that "No words can effectively convey a non-judgmental attitude if the worker does not possess it interiorly" (p. 98).

Earlier we identified that one of the chief anxieties clients experience as they come for help, whether voluntarily or under external pressure, is the fear of being judged. This chapter will focus primarily on the need for sensitivity to this anxiety as we fulfill our professional responsibility. This includes our making appropriate judgments of the behavior, but not of the person, in the context of assessment, as a basis for planning work toward the resolution of the clients' problems.

THE THINKING
AND FEELING COMPONENTS

As we begin practice we need to work through very carefully the difficulty we may initially have in accepting the nonjudgmental attitude as integral to helping and making it a part of ourselves as we grow in our helping capacities. This requires that we examine the meaning of the principle within our own scale of standards and values. Biestek suggests that there are three guidelines to help us in this process.

First, we all approach life with our own standards and values. These are necessary to each of us as guides in our beliefs, our actions, and our interactions with others. Furthermore, we all have responsibility for the kind of society in which we live, and we cannot abandon this as we enter professional practice.

Second, clients are not helped if we appear indifferent to antisocial or illegal behavior, or values that have gotten them into trouble. Particularly in child protection, probation, and parole, and working with sex offenders, effective help consists of helping these clients to accept the reality of society's basic expectations and—it is to be hoped—incorporate them as values of their own (Siporin, 1975:65).

Third, implementing this principle does not mean that the worker must abandon his or her own standards and values. We need to hold on to them, but we must not insist that they are necessarily the right code for all our clients (Biestek, 1957:94-95). The nonjudgmental attitude is an important tool in creating the safe environment in which clients can feel free to talk about their troubles, as they perceive and feel them. We need to be on guard against allowing our own convictions to load our assessment of whether our clients' values are right or wrong. Our prime concern must always be whether or not these values work for or against the clients' psychosocial functioning and well-being.

Neisser suggests that many parents have given unclear and inconsistent instruction to their children about the level of importance of various values, along a continuum from those vitally significant for social living to rules which, while their observance is desirable, are of lesser importance (1965:279). This can mean that their children reach adulthood with a tendency to live with a vague sense of condemnation, ranging from a diffuse sense of inadequacy to severe, unspecified feelings about being "bad." (Neisser, 1965:281)

The nonjudgmental attitude must be made explicit to clients early in the contact. We can do this if we are alert to cues that indicate they are anticipating being judged and blamed. We can clarify that we are evaluating behavior and not the person. We also need to be careful that we do not jump to assign guilt or blame to others in the client's situation. This will only confirm their anxious anticipation that the assignment of guilt and blame is integral to the counseling process. Indeed, we often see clients in a marital struggle who initially come with the express purpose of having us determine "who's right and who's wrong."

An exception to the rule of not assigning blame to others is when we are faced with a child or adult victim of sexual abuse. Irrational self-blame is integral to these persons' struggles, and in these cases, from the beginning of contact, responsibility must be clearly placed with the perpetrator, where it appropriately belongs. This will be discussed in more detail later.

Explicit clarification of this principle will help to free clients to begin to talk openly about their difficulties and to accept responsibility for those aspects of the problem that seem to result from their behavior. While this is particularly applicable in child protection and probation or parole services, it applies equally in the wide variety of difficulties in relationships presented by clients who seek social work services voluntarily. Clients need to express their thoughts and feelings, and they can only feel free to do this as they begin to believe that the worker is not judging them as "a bad person" or "wrong" to have such problems, thoughts, and feelings.

In the political climate at this time of writing I believe this can be especially crucial for workers in income maintenance services. Writing in the 1950s, Biestek stated that "Need rather than 'worthiness' has come to be accepted as the criterion for eligibility for service" (1957:91). As a society, I believe we are in danger of turning back the clock in this matter. The view is becoming prevalent that all people on social assistance of any kind are lazy, do not want to work, cheat the system, and irresponsibly have more children in order to qualify for larger allowances. While some measure of this view has existed in the general population for many years, it appears that in the late 1990s it is beginning to influence social policy. We risk becoming once more a society that stigmatizes those who require welfare services as deficient in moral fiber.[1]

This means that clients who come for any kind of service connected with social assistance come not only with the humiliation of needing such assistance through the loss of unemployment and steady income, the anticipated difficulty of managing on a low fixed income, or with parent-child relationship problems—but also carrying the added burden of public condemnation for not being employed, tax-paying, upstanding citizens. Workers in these areas of practice need to be careful that they do not subscribe to such glib generalizations and that they make their position clear to their clients.

Periodically, public pressures arise that can influence us to condemn certain categories of people and their behavior. We must be on guard and maintain our professional perspective against the "bandwagon" effect of such waves of public hysteria and ill will.

THE RISKS OF PRAISE

Biestek suggests that praise and approval are also subtle forms of judgment and may give clients the impression that they are accepted only conditionally. Clients may then feel they must "stay in the good graces of the social worker" (1957:92-93). We need to bear in mind that both praise and blame

> may have the same effect on the client: to urge him to *hide part of himself.* (1957:93, emphasis added)

Recognizing the clients' strengths can be an important part of therapy, but we need to balance it with a nonjudgmental recognition of weaknesses and areas of difficulty. Neisser makes the significant point that in recognizing both the client's strengths and weaknesses "the client is reassured that he is genuinely accepted, not flattered" (1965:282).

Another result of inappropriate stress on strengths is shown in the following:

At the first meeting of a group of five men and women—adult children of alcoholics—the members were invited to circle in by talking in turn about what was mainly troubling them. The worker, Richard, briefly acknowledged each one's struggle. Knowing that all were employed full-time (they had only been able to attend an evening meeting), he then asked each to tell what they did for a living and how they had reached their present status.

Impressed with how these young men and women had managed to achieve their present positions in spite of their troubled backgrounds, he praised the many good choices they had all clearly made along the way, the good sense they had shown in some instances in limiting contact with their parents, and so on. Richard's intention was genuine; he wanted these men and women to give themselves credit for what they had achieved.

He was surprised to note that the body posture and facial expressions of three members of the group seemed to register anger, and he asked Sally if she was feeling angry. Sally said she was, and Ken and Andy agreed. Richard asked them what it was that had made them angry, and Sally said, "I felt you were saying my pain wasn't anything very much." Ken said it reminded him of his alcoholic father's often repeated accusation: "What have you got to cry about? You've got a warm bed, three square meals, etc, etc."

Richard apologized to the group and tried to explain why he had elaborated on their achievements as a way of helping them feel good about themselves. He said he certainly did not intend to minimize their distress. The group seemed to accept his explanation, but at the close of the meeting Ken and Andy, the two men who had spoken about their anger, said they would not be coming back. They did not think the group could help them. Richard found it hard to understand where he had gone wrong with this group.

Discussion

In attempting to help the group members hold on to good feelings about how they had come this far out of such troubled backgrounds, this worker had, it seemed to his clients, overstressed these aspects of their lives. In discussion with his supervisor it became clear that during the first circling in he had spent a much longer time on this than he had on recognizing their pain and distress.

Together they also looked at his timing. Was it really appropriate, at the first meeting, to devote so much time to their achievements? As Richard had introduced himself and explained the purposes of the group, he had told the members that this was a place where they could talk freely—many of them for the first time—about what they were struggling with in coming to terms with the pain and disappointments of their troubled childhoods.

Richard came to see that they needed to feel that he truly was listening and hearing them. The kind of commendation that would have been appropriate near the close of the first meeting would have been simply to endorse their decision to join the group, as a good first step in working toward change in their lives and relationships.

As it was, at least three group members had interpreted Richard's commendation as "blame"—a negative judgment, perhaps about their inability to put their unhappy memories behind them. The plus side for this worker was that, after observing their nonverbal response, he explored their anger with them undefensively. This is a good example of how clients can teach us about how to help them, if we are strong enough to give them the opportunity and they are strong enough to express their feelings.

RISKS OF ADVICE-GIVING

Another aspect of the importance of the nonjudgmental attitude in the early stages of intervention is suggested by Neisser, who says that clients often "initially see help as asking for and receiving advice." She reminds us that

> we must guard against the indirect judgment implicit in the giving of premature and unsolicited advice. (1965:280)

Giving unsolicited advice implies hasty judgment and distorts the worker-client relationship, setting us up as the expert with quick and easy answers. Those of us who have experienced this kind of reaction after sharing a problem with a friend recall that it conveyed a demeaning implication that "if you were as smart as me you'd have thought of that yourself." This is not only unhelpful, it is actively damaging to persons who come to us in a vulnerable state.

The Feeling Component

Self-awareness is one of the keys to our developing an inner sense of feeling and owning the nonjudgmental attitude. Biestek recommends the use of self-awareness (in the sense of introspection), relating our own thoughts, feelings, and actions to our study of human behavior. He is convinced that

> all knowledge of the dynamics of human nature will remain purely intellectual, academic, static and doubtfully useful . . . unless it is confirmed and tested, . . . through a healthy introspection. (1957:97)

Introspection about how we feel when we are judged will help us to understand clients' anxiety, and to listen attentively and respond sensitively to their struggles.

JUDGMENTS AS PART OF THE ASSESSMENT

It is necessary that we make judgments about the problems clients bring to us, as a basis for appropriate intervention planning. But Neisser says that

> [it is] implicit in the non-judgmental attitude that workers be aware they cannot make a valid diagnostic assessment on brief acquaintance. (1965:280)

By a hasty summation and/or interpretation of the clients' problems, we give the impression of jumping to conclusions, when clients know that there is more they want and need to tell us once their trust in us becomes more secure. Clients are not impressed by our "cleverness" in this way. On the contrary, they may find us shallow and in a hurry to get down to business, or as noted above, they may fear losing our approval.

The second effect of a hurried "diagnosis" after hearing few facts is that we distort the worker-client roles by depriving clients of a sense that we believe they can contribute to the process of therapeutic change (Neisser, 1965:281). In discussing empowerment and the importance of involving clients fully in the helping process, we shall see that it is vital that we recognize that *they* are the experts about their troubles, their life events, and their beliefs, attitudes, and feelings. Hasty diagnostic judgments give the opposite impression, and the distortion of roles contributes to any feelings a client may have that we will bring about the desired change without their help. This is contrary to the objectives of "help" as social work defines them.

Another form of unintentional "judgment" is cited by Biestek, who reminds us of the risk involved in telling clients of similar troubles experienced by others. He says that

> this gives the client the impression of being put in a category. Classification represents a type of judgment. (1957:99)

This matter of premature categorization carries also the danger that it can close our minds to further information, because we may feel we have a complete and satisfactory assessment. It may also have the "filtering" effect discussed earlier, in tempting us to block out new information that does not "fit" our classification. With these risks in mind, there is some professional debate about the use of the currently popular *DSM (Diagnostic and Statistical Manual of Mental Disorders)* scales in assessment. Certainly there is a place for classification in practice, but we need to be careful that it is always undertaken for the client's benefit, and not for the professional's convenience.

Judgments about Others' Actions

As noted above, victims of childhood sexual abuse, regardless of their age when they begin to share the experience with us, characteristically carry a heavy load of self-blame. With these clients we need to make it perfectly clear that we, and any other responsible persons in our society, see the responsibility for the abuse as resting solely with the perpetrator, and that their self-blame is not by any standards valid.

It is particularly important to alleviate self-blame with those clients who recognize and admit that in spite of not wanting the sex act, they sometimes experienced some physical pleasure (depending on their age at the time and the behavior of the perpetrator). Someone has written that these people hate the fact that "their physiology betrayed them."[2] They need help to accept that their physiological response did not make them "bad." It was simply beyond their control and must not be used as a weapon of self-blame.

In cases in which a close family member was the abuser, we need to assign responsibility clearly but without totally condemning the person. In my own experience I have found that adult victims disclosing the abuse for the first time become anxious about being closely related to such a "bad person." They may ask themselves the haunting question, "How can I feel good about myself, coming from a 'sick' family?" This is a question that we often see in clients with other types of dysfunctional family histories.

The nonjudgmental approach is a challenge for most of us, as we listen to how some children have been seduced by a father or older brother with protestations of "special love"; how their silence has been bought with gifts that were skillfully geared to their particular needs and wishes. It is hard to control our justifiable anger as we hear of a nine-year-old boy repeatedly raped by an older brother and his friends, or a neglected little girl being sexually abused by her grandmother, the only person the child felt really cared about her. And we can find ourselves enraged by the mother who clearly knew about the abuse, but ignored or rejected the child's reporting and did nothing about it.

Joining the clients in expressions of rage against others is not helpful. We may appear to be judging others of whose life circumstances we know nothing. Clients will sense this even while they want to know it is safe for them to express their feelings. We need to control our rage, so that we can help clients express their anger. We can acknowledge that we share it, but in a composed way.[3] Thus we can objectively assign responsibility appropriately where it belongs.

When these cases come to us while criminal charges are still legally possible, we need to support society's judgment that these matters should come to trial and thus reenforce the correct responsibility theme with the client. But in many instances these experiences are only brought to us many years after the abuse took place, often even after the death of the person who committed the acts. This places the onus on us to make society's position clear to the client on where the responsibility lies for such acts.

Clients who are struggling with anger about being shortchanged in childhood by the inadequacies of their parents often feel guilty about their resentments and are anxious about expressing their anger. A nonjudgmental approach from us helps these clients. If we accept their right to be angry at what they were not given, over time we can help them accept that, for example, their mother's overwhelming need for the financial security of father's paycheck took precedence over the children's needs.

Where the facts support such an assessment of emotional deprivation, I have found that it helps to offer such clients the view that their parents simply did not have the capacity to be what British psychiatrist David Winnicott has called "good-enough" parents. As noted earlier, this is making a valid judgment about behavior, not a wholesale condemnation of the person, and it seems to be acceptable to troubled adult children in recovery.

We cannot establish the nonjudgmental attitude within us at a certain stage of our professional development and then take it for granted as permanently "ready-to-hand," so to speak (Biestek, 1957:98). To some extent, each new client or group of clients may challenge our commitment to the principle—by unappealing factors in how they present themselves, in their apparent approach to life or to their difficulties (Neisser, 1965:278), or when they report such abhorrent examples of others' behavior as those cited above. Our helping abilities will depend on continual, vigilant self-awareness—recognizing what kinds of judgments we are inwardly making, and in the process guarding against breaching this principle.

SUMMARY OF MAIN POINTS

1. The nonjudgmental attitude is a key value principle in the helping relationship for professional social workers.
2. All clients who come to us for service, for whatever reason, are entitled to our exercise of the nonjudgmental attitude by right of their human individuality.

3. Our professional responsibility requires us to make judgments of behavior, not of the person, and these judgments are made in the context of assessment and intervention planning, never of assigning blame or guilt.
4. We have a social responsibility to uphold with our clients the legal and moral standards and values governing public safety and respect for persons and property in our society.
5. We need not abandon our own personal standards and values, but must not insist that they are the right code for everyone, including our clients.
6. This attitude must be made explicit to clients early in the contact, and reiterated when we see their anxiety about being judged resurfacing.
7. Clients may interpret praise as a judgment, and this can exacerbate their anxiety about not "measuring up" to our standards.
8. We must be careful not to buy into any politically popular classifications of groups of persons as "unworthy" of respect and full professional service.
9. A hasty statement of assessment, or an early offering of advice, gives the client the feeling that we are making a quick judgment on the basis of incomplete information. The disrespect inherent in this implies that we do not have time to hear them out.
10. When clearly assigning to others their responsibility for damaging behavior that has affected our clients, it is important that we do not come across as condemning the person.
11. Self-awareness and healthy introspection are the keys to making the nonjudgmental attitude an integral element of our practice.

NOTES

1. See Siporin (1975: 64-65) for some background discussion of this.
2. I have been unable to trace this quote.
3. We can release our rage later, either when we are alone, or with a trusted colleague.

REFERENCES

Biestek, Felix P. (1957). *The Casework Relationship*. Chicago, IL: Loyola University Press.

Neisser, Marianne. (1965). "Judgments and the Non-Judgmental Attitude in Therapeutic Relationships." *Social Casework*, 46(5):278-282.

Siporin, Max. (1975). *Introduction to Social Work Practice*. New York: Macmillan Publishing Company, Inc.

Chapter 8

Controlled Emotional Involvement: The Disciplined Use of Self as Instrument

Controlled emotional involvement is another essential component of the worker's disciplined use of self as instrument in the helping relationship. It has three elements: empathic sensitivity, guided by cognitive understanding, in the service of the therapeutic purpose (Biestek, 1957:50-60).

Controlled emotional involvement may be defined as:

> The empathic sensitivity of the worker to the client's feelings, disciplined by self-awareness, such that the worker's feelings do not inappropriately affect his or her understanding and purposeful response.

We need to distinguish between empathy and sympathy. We need to feel genuinely and deeply with–but not like–our clients. We must not allow our empathy to become confused by an overflow of feelings of our own that do not belong in the clients' and our shared, here-and-now purpose in the helping relationship.

This confusion can arise, as earlier stated, either as overidentification, or, in the sense of losing respect for the client, as what might be termed "underidentification." It may also arise where feelings stemming from our own current or past experience are triggered by something in the clients' situation itself, or by their feelings about or approach to an event in their lives.

In overidentification, we may lose sight of the therapeutic purpose and inappropriately make allowances for a client who has triggered an emotional response in us that is sympathetic, rather than empathic.

Joel, a worker new to a residential setting for troubled adolescents, had formed a sound working relationship with Brian, a fourteen-year-old boy placed in the facility by child welfare court order. Brian had a history of sexual abuse by his stepfather, had later experimented with drugs, refused to go to school, and lastly did some rather minor shoplifting, which seemed to the child welfare agency to be a "cry for help"–perhaps for external control.

Brian was a spunky, amusing boy, and Joel felt he had been making a real effort to control his foul language and his fighting with other boys. These young people knew at all times their status on demerit points for breaking rules, and that accumulating a certain number would disqualify them for privileges. These might be attending an on-site movie or going home for the weekend, and so on. Brian, due to go home for the first time for a weekend (his stepfather was no longer in the home), had racked up more demerits than the allowable score, and Joel had to tell him that the visit home must be cancelled.

Joel felt that some of the other guys had been "baiting" Brian in the past two weeks. Before telling Brian about the cancellation, he discussed with the residence director whether an exception could be made in his case, because of some improvement and the other boys' aggravations.

Discussion

This is a classic instance of a lack of controlled emotional involvement. This worker's own feelings were involved because some aspects of Brian's personality strongly appealed to him. Perhaps he admired this boy's spunk and humor in the face of so many tough life experiences. Perhaps also the sexual abuse triggered an anger which, while readily understandable, had led him to take sides with Brian in some of his everyday struggles in the cottage. He was overidentifying with this client.

The purpose of the setting was therapeutic work with these young people, to help them change their attitudes, beliefs, and behavior. Integral to the program were unvarying and clearly known consequences, rewards for prosocial, and deprivation of privileges for antisocial behavior. The worker's feelings for this youngster got in the way of what Brian needed to learn–people who care about you can enforce the rules fairly and consistently because they care about you and about helping you to straighten out your life.

The case also illustrates that effective help to this client required that the worker keep his feelings always in balance with his knowledge, his understanding, and the therapeutic purpose (Biestek, 1957:58).

THE DANGER OF TAKING SIDES

This case also touches on another aspect of the difficulty of controlling our emotional involvement–the importance of not taking one client's side over another's, especially when there are diverse views of the problem and how to resolve it in a family, or in a community group or organization.

This can be difficult for us because our own feelings can inhibit our full acceptance of each and every individual client as they present themselves to us. As indicated earlier, some of our clients may have attributes that are unappealing at first contact, and which may persist over a period of time. We must be aware of our inner response to such a person, and ensure that we do not come across as rejecting and lacking in understanding. Without such attention to our own feelings, we may, for example, take sides between family members and unwittingly negate the value of the family therapy method, or undermine our effectiveness in a community practice setting.

> A group of residents in a low-income neighborhood got together with the idea of starting a drop-in center for new mothers and babies. They called an open meeting and, with a well-organized phone campaign, got twenty-three women to attend.
>
> There was some good discussion about what was needed to get things under way. Various approaches clearly had to be made at the outset. The local health services had to be asked if they would provide part-time nursing advice; some local churches or the school board had to be approached about providing accommodation for the program, hopefully rent-free. The group felt that they needed to develop a clear Mission statement and a description of what was to be offered, so that women invited to attend the center could know its general purpose and how it could benefit them.

Four women volunteered to form a committee to get things started. This was accepted by the group. As things began to move along, Marilyn, a community worker with the department of social services, was approached for help by two of the original group members. Kathleen and Gina described how the interested women in the community were becoming divided about the way things were going. They explained their fear that the project might be destroyed unless something was done to get things back on track.

The main difficulty seemed to be that a majority of the original movers were feeling that the volunteers who had taken on the committee work had "taken over" the project. It was felt that they were making decisions among themselves about planning issues, and that the neighborhood women were never brought together for information, or given the chance to discuss how this or that move might work.

There seemed to be some feeling that the four women who had volunteered for the committee were from the "better-off" families in the neighborhood. This had exacerbated the feelings of the others that the committee was not taking into account the right of the whole group to participate in the planning and decision making.

When Kathleen and Gina and two of their friends tried to bring these feelings to the committee members, the latter took great offense. They accused the group of not appreciating all the time and effort the committee had put in, and they threatened to cancel the basic planning that had been started and to withdraw from the project altogether.

Kathleen and Gina felt that this could be disastrous. Not only would it be very hard to start over, but they felt, with some justice, that it would affect the reputation of the project itself vis-à-vis community bodies–municipal, school, church groups–whose support was needed in many practical ways.

Marilyn's own background was from a poor family whose income was social assistance. With the encouragement of her single mother and an older brother, she had completed school and worked her way through college. She remembered painful experiences in high school, where the attitudes of some of the "rich kids" were humiliating to poor youngsters, in matters of clothes, leisure interests, vacation plans, and so on.

Her first inclination was definitely to sympathize with Kathleen and Gina, but, after examining where this feeling came from, she realized that it did not belong in this situation, in which she had a professional helping responsibility. In discussion with her supervisor, Marilyn recognized that to be helpful she needed to accept and feel with both parties in this dispute.

Her first interview with the project committee clearly showed that their distress was genuine. They had indeed worked hard, used some of their personal networks effectively, and had made some good progress in initial planning. They had called two meetings to discuss their moves with the general neighborhood group, but a very poor turnout both times had given them the feeling that such discussion was not really needed. They had decided not to call any more general meetings until final decisions needed the group's ratification. They were hurt and upset at the reaction this had caused.

Marilyn learned that they had set both these meetings at dates and times to suit themselves. At rather short notice they had called only the one or two women they knew best, not the four prime movers, asking them to "let the others know." The committee members now realized that this had not been an effective way to reach the group, and it had resulted in the poor attendance. But to the other group members it had also, unfortunately, given a "cliquey" appearance to the committee's relationship to the group as a whole, and this had been resented.

Marilyn suggested to the committee, and to Kathleen and Gina, that the first step, as she saw it, would be to call a general meeting of all the interested women in order to discuss how to resolve the difficulties that had arisen. She offered to act as "facilitator" for the discussion, to which both groups gratefully agreed. Although one committee member had suggested that they would need a "mediator," Marilyn purposely used the more positive term. She felt that "mediation" might set the stage for people to come to the meeting with the goal of voicing grievances, rather than resolving what seemed to be getting in the way of achieving the group's main purpose.

In discussion with her supervisor, Marilyn realized that being aware of and controlling her own feelings was going to be a critical factor in her role at the general meeting. In her meeting with the committee members, some of the ways two of them expressed their feelings about "the others" had revealed attitudes that triggered old feelings for Marilyn about "rich snobs" vs. ordinary–i.e., poor–people. She had caught herself reacting inwardly with the old angry resentment, but had been able to set those inappropriate feelings aside and to respond to these women's real distress that their hard work was not appreciated.

At the general meeting it was important for Marilyn, in her role as facilitator, to help the group stay focused on their main objective: the drop-in center for new mothers and babies. She suggested that the members formulate their mission statement out loud, even though its final form was not completely set. They could then begin to address what seemed to be getting in the way of realizing their objective.

Circling in then gave each person in turn the chance to express, without interruption or comment, their view of what the difficulties were and to give their ideas for solutions. In this way the group could ultimately "own" the solutions to the problems. The class difference problem was brought out by Gina and another member in this process. Marilyn felt it was good to get this out in the open. A committee member, speaking soon after Gina, handled this very openly and without defensiveness, admitting that perhaps the way they had been handling things had given an "exclusive" impression. She wanted the group to know that they, too, really wanted the drop-in center to succeed.

This enabled Marilyn to draw the group together again by having them emphasize the common theme of their shared objective.

It was useful at that point to examine some of the practical, organizational difficulties. There was clearly a need to establish an effective method for calling meetings. The second issue was that while the committee members felt overworked, the other women felt underinvolved. The committee needed to be expanded and the work needed to be shared more equitably. A more formal structure and designation of responsibilities in the reorganization overall was discussed and agreed upon.

This meeting re-established the cohesiveness of this neighborhood group, and the will to work together for their goal was reaffirmed. Two months later Marilyn received an invitation to the opening ceremony of the Riverview Neighborhood Drop-in Center for New Mothers and Babies. The ceremony was performed the by the neighborhood's municipal representative, herself a new mother.

Discussion

Focusing on this group's prime objective helped the worker as well as the group; it acted as a constant reminder for them all that the class difference was not the issue. Marilyn controlled her emotional inclination to take sides with the low-income group by focusing on helping them all work toward the achievement of their goal.

OTHER PRACTICE AREAS
INVOLVING THIS PRINCIPLE

Any and all fields of practice can present us with difficulty in controlling our emotional involvement, but space requirements limit discussion here to certain selected areas. At the time of this writing, issues of aging and terminal illness, including HIV disease, are involving both family service and medical social workers, and there is much literature on the subject. These clients clearly challenge our implementation of this principle, and they have been chosen for examination here.

Issues of Care for the Elderly and the Terminally Ill

Work with the Aged

Working with these clients can trigger unresolved conflicts for many of us, connected with our relationship with own parents, or fears about our own aging (Sprung, 1989:598).

The first contact for workers in a family service setting is often meeting with a "sandwich-generation" couple who are considering whether or not they need to change the living arrangements of their aging parent(s). This can trigger some of our own feelings about filial duty vs. institutional care, and/or about the adult child's attitude toward the parent–are they approaching this decision with affection and respect or in an uncaring way?

The situation may include the adult child and his or her spouse, and adolescent or young adult children living at home. The worker needs to accept and understand the pertinent reality for each person in this configuration, and to empathize with all parties involved. We need, for example, to watch ourselves for inappropriately feeling protective of the elder where the adult children are seeing institutional care–in spite of the parent's resistance–as the best solution. Sprung suggests that in such a case we may see ourselves as needing to perform a "good child" role that may originate in our relationship to our own parents (1989:600). This may arise where a conflicted relationship to our own parents carries a residue of guilt about having rejected them. Conversely, it might arise from a protective feeling for beloved parents, that "I would *never* put my parent in an old-age home." Either may lead us to put undue pressure on the adult children to care for–or continue caring for–their parent in their own home rather than helping them to make an informed, carefully considered choice about institutional care. Whatever their relationship is to their parent, they will feel judged and blamed. It will also seriously interfere with our giving the elder the kind of help he or she needs in accepting the plan.

Cultural factors may also influence a decision about institutional care, either for the worker or for the family who are considering it for their parent. If institutional care is contrary to our own cultural beliefs, the control of our emotions will lie in our focussing on these clients as individuals facing this decision, within their own cultural framework. If cultural influences are pressuring the clients, our helping role may be to help them reexamine a bias that, taking all their circumstances into account, needs to be reevaluated.

In direct work with the aged, Sprung suggests that some elder clients may react to the worker as if he or she were their child. We do not help these clients if we react to them as if they were our own parent (1989:600). Emotional involvement of this kind can deprive our client of the rights to which they are entitled; the relationship's boundaries become blurred and we can lose sight of our professional responsibility.

In working with some depressed elders we may become enmeshed in the sadness of their losses–of beloved partners, of long-standing friends, of health, independence, mobility, or mental faculties. Sprung points out that we need to be careful that we do not begin to feel "as overwhelmed, frustrated and helpless as the client" (1989:601). This will require our controlled emotional involvement, not just to protect ourselves but to protect the client. We must not let our feelings get in the way of our responsibility to help them face and accept their losses. We need to help them look at the joys they did experience, which nothing can take away from them, and to find ways, however small they may seem, in which they can maintain some control over their lives.

Miss V, aged eighty-four, left her home one year ago to live in a fairly large, multiple-level care residence for the aged, located in a small town near her former home. Several long-time friends had also retired to live there, but since she had arrived three of these had moved into the "partial care" or "total care" areas and two had died. Miss V felt very lonely and increasingly depressed. Jennifer, the resident social worker at the residence, found her visits with Miss V almost overwhelming. The woman's life seemed to have been very narrow. She had never married, and several factors–a good family income, the custom of her generation and social milieu, her parents' possessiveness, and her own lack of initiative–had combined to preclude a career outside the home. She had cared for her parents until they died and lived alone thereafter. She wept a lot during Jennifer's visits, and talked of hoping to die soon, although she was in robust good health for her age, had a good appetite, and showed no symptoms of clinical depression.

Jennifer felt some irritation at Miss V's despondent attitude, and felt that Miss V was "using" her simply as a means of venting her depression. Her attempts to suggest a different approach seemed fruitless and she gradually found "reasons" for postponing regular talks with Miss V, who reproached her occasionally—"I looked for you on Tuesday" and so on. This made Jennifer feel guilty, but still she avoided more frequent contact.

Miss V's nephew lived about two hours away, and he and his wife visited her fairly regularly, but recently there had been longer intervals between their visits. On their most recent visit this couple had asked to see Jennifer privately and had admitted to her that Miss V's gloomy attitude and complaints about almost everything in the residence were very depressing for them. She also reacted with a critical attitude to almost anything they told her about their own lives. For example, they were supporting their eighteen-year-old daughter's carefully thought-out plan to take a year off between high school and college. She was applying for student work in a third world development program. Miss V had "lectured" them about letting Melissa become a "drifter," etc.

Both Mr. V and his wife worked outside the home full-time. One child was away at college, and Melissa and a younger brother were still living at home. They felt guilty that they could not offer Miss V a home with them, but they knew that it would not work. Miss V had lived alone for thirty years and was very set in her ways about housekeeping and so on. They knew Miss V appreciated their visits, and they felt badly that finding these so stressful was making it easy for them to find reasons to postpone them.

After this interview Jennifer realized that the couple was mirroring her own pattern of relating to Miss V, and that she was allowing her own feelings to get in the way of fulfilling her professional responsibility to this client. During her next visit, Jennifer got Miss V to talk about her early life on a family farm in the area. She talked interestingly about her childhood, walking to school through "mountains of snow," chores, a fire in the family's barn, and so on.

Jennifer called the nephew and suggested that during their visits they talk with Miss V about her memories and ask her to let them tape these for them and their children. This reminded Mr. V that when they helped her clear out her house, she had given them a box of old family photographs, but none had names or dates on them. He suggested that they would bring these on one of their visits and get her to name them, as she was the only person still living who knew who these people were.

From time to time, a local church would bring to the residence large flower arrangements, donated by a bereaved family following a funeral. Miss V had always thought that these flowers were poorly arranged around the residence, and, passing the utility room one morning and seeing a volunteer arranging them in small vases for various locations, she offered to help. As a result she was regularly called upon for this task, for which she had a real flair. It gave her a sense of being needed and, since she assisted in wheeling the filled vases to various locations around the residence, she was often welcomed and commended by residents and staff for her "way with arranging flowers."

Gradually Miss V's mood improved. Her nephew and his wife, sometimes joined by two of their children, genuinely enjoyed her memories, and Miss V enjoyed hearing some of it played back to her on tape. They told Jennifer that giving names to the photographs had led to amusing stories about family eccentrics and some early pioneering adventures–stories that had been handed down over several generations. Miss V began to feel valued in the family because her memories were something only she could offer them. This, and the recognition she received for arranging flowers, gave her a renewed feeling of self-worth and some capacity for influence. She began to focus on what she had to offer others, and this helped to relieve her previous preoccupation with sadness and loss.

Discussion

In the process of accepting, understanding, and responding to the feelings of the concerned relatives, this worker's self-awareness helped her to examine her own reaction to this client. She was able to identify the feelings of irritation and helplessness that were getting in the way of her offering any effective help to Miss V By accepting these feelings, without defensiveness, she was able to explore previously untapped possibilities to help Miss V reclaim a more positive sense of herself and of having the potential to influence even a small part of the structure of her life at this stage.

Erikson's Theory of Personality Development in Aging

Erikson's delineation of age-stage ego-tasks provide one way of examining the elder's difficulty at a crucial milestone in his or her life. In his view, mental health in old age consists in accepting that the whole of one's life, as it was lived, is our own responsibility. It could not have been different, in his view, because of who we were, and the choices we made at each stretch of the road (1980: 104-105). This level of acceptance requires that in old age we do not judge ourselves or others harshly for what has not been experienced or achieved and that we let go of bitterness and useless regrets about "what might have been."

As social workers offering services to elders at this stage of their life, we need to accept and empathize with those who are trapped in the negative response–Erikson's "despair and disgust." We need to be very much aware of our own feelings and where they come from, as we listen to what perhaps sounds to us like a life story in which it seems that personal rigidity and/or bitterness influenced many choices that resulted in unmet needs and unhappiness. Do our feelings come from some unresolved conflicts in our relationship to our own parents? Perhaps we are comparing the missed opportunities that this still physically healthy client had for a full and rewarding life, with our own beloved grandparent who has struggled for the last fifteen years with a debilitating illness for which there is no cure.

When we identify and control our feelings with these clients, we shall be able to understand that the task of accepting and integrating one's life story in old age is rarely easy, and harder for some elders than others. In addition, we shall be better able to help each client face and resolve tasks, not as we want them to, but as they feel able to.

Care of the Terminally Ill

The last twenty-five years have brought many new concepts, in both medical and psychosocial aspects of care for the terminally ill.

Hospice or palliative care, offered in the home and/or hospital settings—some of these being separate facilities so designated—is changing the traditional roles of terminally ill patients, their medical caregivers, and social work services.

The majority of persons with a terminal illness, regardless of their age, are now told of their condition and are given a realistic prognosis, based on the best available medical knowledge. They are also generally given more of an opportunity now to have a say in what kinds of treatment interventions they wish to receive or refuse. Rusnack, Schaefer, and Moxley state that the focus of all caregivers in palliative care is on facilitating what has been called a "safe passage" into death for the patient (1988:3-20).

In a later work, the same authors approach the needs of the terminally ill person in a caring environment using Germain and Gitterman's (1980) thesis that psychosocial health requires a "good-enough fit" between personal needs and resources, and environmental nurture and support. They state that

> The match between the patient and the caring environment of the hospice is enhanced where the self-esteem of patients remains strong, their stage of development is respected, and where the social environment shows an openness to a consideration of the patient's ability to be a coparticipant in the care process. (1991:98)

Lattanzi suggests that "Enhancing the quality of life for dying patients and their families is the essence of hospice care" (cited in Corr and Corr, 1983:229).

Coping with the Stress of Palliative Care

While many of our clients with terminal illness will be in the older age groups, cancer and HIV/AIDS may involve our working in palliative care settings with much younger persons, including children. Many of the issues involved in facing death are the same for patients regardless of their age, but some are unique to the young person, and particularly to the person dying of AIDS. Social workers must take account of how these factors affect their own feelings in taking responsibility for professional help to these patients and their families.

Knowing that an elder client is close to death can stimulate strong and painful feelings for workers that may stem from earlier experiences of loss in their own life. The worker's capacity to identify those feelings and their origin, bringing them into conscious awareness, is critical in helping persons facing death and their families facing bereavement (Pilsecker, 1979:370). Sprung says that in order to be helpful ". . . workers must do effective grief work themselves and acknowledge their own feelings and fears" (1989:599). Lattanzi states that in order to prevent these feelings from blocking our helpfulness,

> one to two years need to have passed [after a worker's bereavement], and the worker needs to have dealt with the loss before undertaking the demands of hospice work. (cited in Corr and Corr, 1983:228)

Most writers in this area emphasize that palliative care workers in all disciplines must take care to plan activities away from work that will maintain their own inner strength (Rusnack, Schaefer, and Moxley, 1988; Vachon, 1979; Pilsecker, 1979).

Pilsecker lists the following fundamental issues with which the social worker must deal as he or she faces this area of practice:

- personal reactions to death
- personal reactions to cancer
- the ability to tolerate uncertainty (1979:370-371)

First, as noted above, we must address our own fears about death. This author suggests that the crucial question to be answered is that of our ability to manage our fears and anxiety in the presence of death while retaining our respect for the person who moves ever closer to it.

Second, the symptoms of late-stage cancer are distressing, and not only in a psychological sense. As Pilsecker points out "sights and smells and sometimes twisted sounds" (1979:370) emanate from the dying patient. These manifestations of suffering can be oppressive for us, knowing that there is nothing we–often anyone–can do to change or relieve the condition. We may also need to realize that some of our difficulty is that we dread cancer for ourselves and for those we love. When the cancer begins to affect the patient's mental functioning, we must be prepared to "sift through the confusion of words and phrases" (1979:370) that the patient may communicate.

Third, there is the uncertainty about the course of the disease. Some patients survive–against all odds–a certain stage of the cancer's development, or a "last resort" line of treatment. Others may die unexpectedly where medical assessment predicted a remission. There is also, as this author reminds us, the "ambiguity of the patient's emotional state" (1979:371). Pilsecker's experience indicates that despite the well-accepted Kübler-Ross five-stage schema that moves the patient through denial, anger, bargaining, depression to acceptance,

> . . . patients have a knack for disrupting any schema, flitting from one emotion to another, challenging us to dare to discard our neat conceptualizations and find out what their feelings really are. (1979:371)

Pilsecker's experience indicates that this ambiguity may arise in connection with the person's readiness to die. At the time of writing some jurisdictions have legislation validating medical acceptance of "Do not resuscitate" orders, living wills, and other formats that allow the patient to make a written statement that nothing should be done to prolong an inevitable and imminent death. Where no legal processes are in force, these statements are often accepted in a voluntary format and acted upon by doctors and the patient's family. Pilsecker cites one case where the patient clearly expressed ambiguity–"I want to die" and "I don't want to die [yet]"–although he had been emphatic about his "Do not resuscitate" order (1979:371). We need to accept and support the patient during these shifts of emotion.

Pilsecker further points out that in deciding when and how to talk to patients about their death, we must be alert to determine whether it is our need to talk about death or theirs. Our training conditions us to opt for the helpful effects of getting feelings out in the open, but we must respect each person's individual right to cope with facing death in the way that works for them. We need to "listen carefully to what the patient tells us," respond to hints of feelings that they do express, and offer comments that open the way, but do not press for further expression of feelings (1979:374-375).

The same author emphasizes the importance of our not trying to influence the patient or their family toward Kübler-Ross' desired resolution of "acceptance." For some people that will be the chosen and workable path. But for others, Dylan Thomas' "Rage, rage, against the dying of the light" may be the strategy that works for them. We may have a personal preference in one direction or the other. Pilsecker says that we need to

> . . . bring the belief clearly into view and consciously root it out of what goes on between you and the client. (1979:373)

The Influence of Religious Beliefs

One further aspect of our emotional involvement in this situation requires our concerned attention to self-awareness. This is the question of religious beliefs and affiliations, particularly the question of belief in an afterlife. We cannot assume that our client shares either our religious faith or the security we may have found without such beliefs. To make ourselves feel better about their death, we may slip into using our own convictions and put pressure on the client as they begin to express either convictions or doubts. They may then follow our lead because of an implied "should" in our communication, which has not left them free to pursue their own line of thinking and questioning. Some clients will want to discuss these issues with a clergyman of their own faith, but we must be careful not to recommend this until we are sure it is what this person really wants. Some who are questioning a religious belief may specifically need to struggle with their uncertainties themselves, perhaps feeling safe to do so with us, rather than with a pastor (Pilsecker, 1979:377-378).

These questions can perhaps be especially poignant for workers in medical settings caring for children and young people facing terminal illness. For many of us the "why?" of these instances is unanswerable.

Care of Terminally Ill Children and Young People

Those who choose to work in palliative care with terminally ill children must carefully assess their ability to cope with the stress of what one writer has called "A Social Worker's Agony" (Priddy, 1990). We need to ensure that our own feelings do not get in the way of the help that the child, the parents, and siblings will all need as they move through the painful process of their family member's approaching death. This level of stress will require our concerned attention to the availability and use of support systems for our own well-being already outlined above.

Palliative Care with HIV Disease Patients

Mount Sinai (Toronto) Hospital's guide on this subject stresses the importance of the personal support network for workers in palliative care with persons with HIV disease (1995:150). Social workers considering this field of practice must examine, perhaps with professional help, their feelings about the disease, and their ability to accept the kind of stress involved in being constantly with persons (often young) whose lives are cut short by a deadly disease. It is true that many people do live longer with HIV than their doctors forecast for them, but at the time of writing research has yielded little hope for a cure.

We need to examine our own feelings about how these patients have contracted this disease. The causes may be varied: shared needles by substance abusers, unprotected sex with a same-sex or opposite-sex partner who did not disclose his or her positive HIV reading, or a tainted blood transfusion.

It will be vital that we recognize what our feelings are about the cause. Some workers will need to seek counseling about their own homophobia. Others will need to face their negative feelings about family members who blame the client for his or her lifestyle as being the cause. We must ensure that these feelings do not interfere with our offering appropriate help to clients and their families. We can accept and share the distress and anger of these deeply troubled clients, but we must not allow *any* personal feelings to dominate what we can offer in constructive help to patient and family as they live with the painful reality of their illness.

We must also recognize that some gay men who contract HIV (and their families) may be coping with a backlog of unresolved issues about their sexuality. Our own feelings about the effects of these coping mechanisms—coming out to some relatives and friends but not to others, for instance—must be kept under careful control as these issues arise. We need to recognize the validity, for each individual, of *their* way of dealing with their own perceived reality.

The list of suggestions that follows gives sound advice for the guidance of workers in controlling their feelings and maintaining their readiness to be truly with, and helpful to these clients as they learn to live with their disease and its inevitable result. Since many of these patients live—and die—at home and are in a hospital or hospice only intermittently, these suggestions are also useful for workers in supporting the patient's family and volunteer caregivers.

The recommendations are that caregivers:

- avoid excessive involvement, which may preclude objective counseling, advice, and medical care;
- recognize that anger directed at the caregiver should not be taken personally, but may be part of the person's coping strategy or the effect of the disease;
- do not allow AIDS care to dominate their life;
- have personal insight into the need for overwork/overinvolvement;
- recognize that immersion in caregiving, both in personal and professional roles, may lead to emotional exhaustion and burnout; and
- realize that maintaining a positive attitude in the face of random suffering promotes coping by enhancing self-esteem and a sense of power. (Ferris et al., 1995:150)

The control of our emotional involvement with our clients in whatever setting we choose to work is an essential factor in whether or not we are truly helpful. It is not an easy skill to learn. It draws on empathy, self-awareness, understanding, and attention to the therapeutic purpose, and is integral to the disciplined use of self in the helping relationship.

SUMMARY OF MAIN POINTS

1. Control of our emotional involvement requires that we distinguish between feeling genuinely with our client (empathy) and feeling like them (sympathy).
2. Overidentification with a client is the unhelpful result of our becoming emotionally caught up in their plight, rather than maintaining our objectivity and therapeutic responsibility.
3. Underidentification arises when personal feelings diminish our respect for the client and inhibit our capacity for empathy.
4. Taking sides in the clients' struggle demonstrates a lack of controlled emotional involvement.
5. The key to controlled emotional involvement is the conscious identification of our feelings and where they come from. This prevents them from getting in the way of the client's needs.
6. Working with elder clients and their families about appropriate care questions may trigger feelings about unresolved issues from our own family that must be recognized and controlled; if they are not controlled, they may block our clients' freedom to choose what they believe is right for them.
7. We must recognize and control our own feelings about death, and about losses through death that we have experienced, to ensure that these do not obscure our hearing our clients' true feelings or those of their family.
8. In hospice or palliative care, we owe it to ourselves and to our clients to maintain a solid support system outside the workplace, so that we do not become overinvolved emotionally to the point of being unable to be helpful.
9. We must be alert not to impose on these clients our own values about facing death, accepting always that they have the right to face it in the individual way that fits their personal needs.
10. We must be prepared to recognize and set aside whatever feelings of our own—anger at the disease itself, at its cause, or frustration about the unanswerable "why?"—that are triggered by working with children and young people who are facing death from any cause.

REFERENCES

Biestek, Felix P. (1957). *The Casework Relationship*. Chicago, IL: Loyola University Press, pp. 48-66.

Corr, Charles A. and Donna M. Corr, eds. (1983). *Hospice Care: Principles and Practice*. New York: Springer Publishing Company.

Erikson, Erik H. (1980). *Identity and the Life Cycle*. New York: W.W. Norton and Company, pp. 104-105.

Germain, Carel B. and Alex Gitterman. (1980). *The Life Model of Social Work Practice*. New York: Columbia University Press.

Lattanzi, Marcia E. (1983). "Learning and Caring: Education and Training Concerns." In *Hospice Care: Principles and Practice*. Corr, Charles A. and Donna M. Corr, eds. New York: Springer Publishing Company, pp. 223-236.

Kübler-Ross, Elisabeth. (1969). *On Death and Dying*. New York: Macmillan.

Mount Sinai Hospital and Casey House Hospice. (1995). *Module 4, Palliative Care: A Comprehensive Guide for the Care of Persons with HIV Disease*. John Flannery, Frank D. Ferris, Helen McNeal, R. Cameron, Gerry Bally, and Michel Morisette, eds. Toronto, Canada: Mt. Sinai Hospital/Casey House Hospice.

Millet, Nina. (1983). "Hospice: A New Horizon for Social Work." In *Hospice Care: Principles and Practice*. Corr, Charles A. and Donna M. Corr, eds. New York: Springer Publishing Company, pp. 135-147.

Pilsecker, Carleton. (1979). "Terminal Cancer: A Challenge for Social Work." *Social Work in Health Care*, 4(4):369-379.

Priddy, Drew. (1990). "A Social Worker's Agony: Working with Children Affected by Crack Cocaine." *Social Work*, 35(3):197-199.

Rusnack, Betty, Sarajane McNulty, and David Moxley. (1988). "Safe Passage: Social Work Roles and Function in Hospice Care." *Social Work in Health Care*, 13(3):3-20.

——— (1991). "Hospice: Social Work's Response to a New Form of Social Caring." *Social Work in Health Care*, 15(2):95-119.

Sprung, Gloria M. (1989). "Transferential Issues in Working with Older Adults." *Social Casework: The Journal of Contemporary Social Work*, 70(10):597-602.

Thomas, Dylan. (1973). "Do Not Go Gentle Into that Goodnight." In Richard Ellman and Robert O'Clair, eds., *The Norton Anthology of Modern Poetry*. New York: W.W. Norton and Co.

Vachon, Mary L.S. (1979). "Staff Stress in Care of the Terminally Ill." *Quality Review Bulletin*, May:13-17. Cited in Corr and Corr. (1983). *Hospice Care: Principles and Practice*. New York: Springer Publishing Company, pp. 238-239.

PART IV:
PRINCIPLES OF METHOD

Chapter 9

Individualization:
Who Are *These* People
and What Is *Their* Trouble?

This principle is one of the most direct expressions in practice terms of the ethical principle of respect for the innate worth and dignity of each human being. As Biestek succinctly puts it,

> It is based upon the right of human beings to be individuals and to be treated not just as *a* human being, but as *this* human being ... (1957:25)

Implementation of this principle in study, assessment, and intervention requires that we continually check to ensure that we are accurately in touch with "who are *these* people, and what is *their* trouble?" Biestek believes that the client's ability to make constructive use of the helping relationship depends directly upon his or her perception of being treated as an individual (1957:27). The client's perception—"I am not just 'another case' to this person"—will require a firm sense of the worker's concerned attention to understanding that the character of the client's struggles reflects that person's unique individuality.

Individualization, as a method principle in social work practice, may be defined as:

> The recognition and understanding that the client's difficulty and pain, while they may be similar to—even shared with—others in the same overall situation, are experienced in ways that are uniquely different to each individual. Effective help will

require that we base all our work firmly upon this premise, and selectively employ differential models, skills and methods in the helping process of study, assessment, and intervention. (adapted from Biestek, 1957:23-27)

NECESSARY CAPACITIES OF THE WORKER

Biestek identifies seven capacities that the worker must have for effective implementation of this principle. These, with some amplifications added, are as follows:

(i) freedom from bias and prejudice, which involves the responsibility for self-awareness;

(ii) knowledge of human behavior, and knowledge of the various ethnic and religious cultures in the community where we work. We need to realize that ". . . knowledge about ethnic minority group life and understanding of the basic dynamics of human behavior are of equal importance if practice is to be effective." (Schlesinger and Devore, 1979:22)

(iii) ability to listen and observe;

(iv) ability to move at the client's pace;

(v) ability to enter into the feelings of people; involving empathy, self-awareness, controlled emotional involvement, and a nonjudgemental attitude;

(vi) ability to keep perspective; involving the ability to see the client(s) in a systemic relationship to his/her/their social environment; and

(vii) flexibility; involving the ability to change objectives and/or methods of intervention in keeping with the clients' developing needs. (adapted from Biestek, 1957:27-30)

Freedom from Bias and Prejudice

As stated earlier, self-awareness is the critical factor in whether or not we can be truly helpful to those who seek or are directed to our services. In paying concerned attention to the individuality of our clients, it is essential that we work to become aware of what unex-amined preconceptions we carry–and may have carried for years.

For example, we may be carrying prejudice against certain cate-gories of persons according to their race, skin color, or ethnic, political, or religious affiliation; a particular trade, profession, or calling; economic status, sexual preference, or a specific personal deficit such as alcoholism, physical violence, or the inability to hold a steady job (Biestek, 1957:27-28). "Prejudice" is an ugly word. Some of our biases may have been so much a part of our habitual mindset that we have never faced up to their true nature. Others may take us by surprise as we begin to work with certain persons or groups of persons, because we may never have had to face a situa-tion that would call them into awareness (Devore and Schlesinger, 1981:83).

The principle of individualization of each and every client will require first that we examine and face such prejudices for what they are, and recognize that these have no place in our professional responsibility for helping people. With this recognition we can begin to see the individuality and unique qualities of this person, family, group, or community as who they are. We can then begin to shed some of the prejudice or bias that may have initially catego-rized them in a derogatory way (Garrett, 1942).

Most of our prejudices are rooted in ignorance. Because we have never actually gotten to know any of the categorized person(s) as individual human beings, the stereotype that has colored our mind-set has not had any infusion of new information that would force us to examine and question its validity. The client-worker relationship– seeing this person as another human being having the right to claim our caring attention–can become the route to enlightenment.

As discussed earlier, other biases may be carryovers from our own childhood. For example, if I was the child of alcoholic parents, seeing the effects of my alcoholic clients' behavior on their children may trigger the troubled child still within me. I need to remind myself that they are who they are, and I am who I am. I must ensure that my adult self is "in charge" of what I feel and do in this situation, not my hurt child. I must not let the old fears, anger, and pain get in the way of meeting my responsibility to help this couple with the difficulty that has brought them to me.

Knowledge of Human Behavior

As indicated earlier, knowledge of human behavior is an integral part of the professional social worker's intellectual equipment. Our essential learning for the understanding of troubled people–whether we meet them as individuals, families, groups, organizations, or communities–is drawn from the disciplines of psychology, psychiatry, sociology, medicine, and philosophy.[1] Social work's task–and unique contribution–is that of putting together, selectively, knowledge from these fields, appropriate in each instance, in order to understand the whole bio-psycho-social reality of our clients and to help them make effective use of the agency's service (Biestek, 1957:28).

We sometimes hear people assert that common sense, life experience, and compassion are more significant than "theory" in helping people in trouble. "Common Sense" in this context can be seriously overrated. It is almost by definition a generalization that has no place in the individualization of each and every person who comes to us in trouble. My clients' view of what is practical and workable for them may have nothing in common with mine, and my view of what is "sensible" for them may make no sense to them at all. Some elements of the public often present "common sense" as a remedy for a particular instance of a social problem. In actuality it masks a "knee-jerk" reaction to the issue, and as such has no place in the considered, holistic approach that is the task of professional social work.

A worker's life experience may be valuable, but we must not assume it is an automatic key to understanding another's feelings. It can be useful as a way of entering into clients' feelings about their situation, but only if we have recognized and accepted it as our own and individual to us. It is not a "recipe" for solving a similar problem for another unique individual. The way one worker faced and survived childhood trauma, the things that motivated another to "kick the habit" of his or her addiction, or the path a third took out of an abusive marriage–all of these experiences may quite simply have no relevance for our client. To offer these, even with the best of intentions, is to deny that person's right to be him or herself. The worker's responsibility for self-awareness will be the safeguard here. We need to recognize that the use of our own experiences may actually be an inappropriate denial of our client's right and need to be understood as a unique individual (Biestek, 1957:28).

Compassion is an indispensable quality in our approach to helping people. Fortunately it is often a major component in our motivation to become social workers. We need to learn to care deeply about the struggles and the pain of everyone in need of our help, the initially off-putting person as well as the more immediately appealing. However, we also have to realize that while caring is necessary, it is by no means a sufficient quality for the effective helping professional. It has to be coupled with knowledge of human behavior and theories of study, assessment, and intervention.

In a course called Theory for Practice, I used to illustrate the risk of compassion without knowledge of theory with the example of the certainly ineffectual–perhaps fatal–results of my incompetence as a swimmer trying to help another swimmer in difficulty, despite my being highly motivated by compassion. I was often lucky enough to have in my classes a qualified Red Cross lifesaver. In contrast to my all-too-compassionate efforts, this student would explain the principles of "Go, (close enough but not within touch); talk calmly; throw (a life belt, towel, or rope); and tow."

This is in effect a "theory" of lifesaving based on sound knowledge of principles of water safety, which would in most instances save the person's life. It was interesting also to discover that this lifesaving practice included a valuable element of involving the troubled person actively in the helping process–while holding on to whatever had come handy for towing, the distressed swimmer was encouraged to paddle with his or her legs as part of the successful towing operation. We also noted a parallel between the maintenance of a certain physical distance–for the safety of both–and the principle of controlled emotional involvement.

In summary, then, life experience can be useful if it is processed through keen self-awareness, and if there is steady adherence to the client's individuality. One's life experience is not an adequate substitute for knowledge of human behavior from the social sciences. Compassion, although essential, is not by itself effective. The warmly compassionate heart must be informed by the cool, knowledgeable head, and the calm, enlightened head needs information from the sensitive, caring heart.

As noted earlier, we need to guard against the danger of using our knowledge of human behavior to categorize, rather than individualize the clients' troubling experience. This will actually obscure what it is that makes an apparently similar experience uniquely different for each person, family, group, or community.[2]

Erikson (1950, 1980) has taught us a great deal about what is common to the experience of adolescence in North American society:

> You are assigned to work in a special school setting with a group of students, aged fifteen to sixteen years, male and female, who have been expelled from regular classrooms for violent behavior. You will of course need to recognize that all these young people are sharing the biological and psychosocial stresses of adolescence in the same community, although they have attended different schools.
>
> However, while you need to recognize their common biological experience, you will not be helpful if you do not take into account that the psychosocial aspects, and in particular the struggle for identity, have very different meanings for the son of the CEO of the local branch of XXY Insurance Co., the daughter of a single mother on social assistance, the son of a black Caribbean immigrant family, the fifteen-year-old struggling with his growing conviction that he is gay, and the daughter of an unemployed Native American couple, recently moved from the reservation into the city's low-rental housing project.

We need to recognize also that this concept of individual difference applies equally to groups of persons. Each family, despite similarities in age, family composition, economic status, ethnic background, etc. will have its own unique patterns of relating, of defining difficulties, dealing with conflict, identifying causes, and solving problems. The same will apply to formed groups, whether their purpose is personal growth or task accomplishment. Each group will demonstrate, as it moves into and becomes a working group with a shared purpose, individual characteristics that make it uniquely different from others having the same purpose.

Likewise, each community or organization will have its own particular characteristics, its way of interrelating, its power structure, its way of dealing with conflict, its own perception of the root causes of the difficulty, and its own approach to problem solving. With each client system we need to select different models, skills, and methods in our practice, tailoring these to the specific needs of each, as they reveal them to us (Biestek, 1957:26).

ETHNIC-SENSITIVE PRACTICE

It is appropriate here to discuss the reality that social workers today can count on working with populations that include persons of different ethnic backgrounds. Gordon defines an ethnic group as consisting ". . . of those people who share a unique social and cultural heritage and a historical past" (1964:513). It is vital for the effective provision of service that we recognize and understand what these shared elements mean to those of ethnic backgrounds different from our own.

In their valuable discussion of what they describe as ethnic-sensitive practice, Devore and Schlesinger point out that:

All clients are a part of two systems. (1) The dominant system which is the source of power and economic resources and (2) the nurturing system, composed of the physical and social environment. (1987:513)

They emphasize that this axiom has special meaning for us when we work with ethnic groups and minorities. Their definition of ethnicity's basic elements states that:

[They are] the associated sense of peoplehood and identification with the group. These include national origin, religion, a common language and race. (1987:513)

Devore and Schlesinger quote other writers in feeling that it is no longer useful to use the term "minority" in a strictly numerical sense. Rather they believe it is logical today to speak of disadvantaged persons as minorities, that is [those people] at the lowest end of the spectrum of power and advantage. (Hopps, 1983-1984:77)

These authors also point out that ethnic sensitive practice needs to be implemented when we are working with any of the disadvantaged groups in our society. These persons, though not necessarily immigrants, frequently share a sense of ethnicity, as it is defined above, with others of their group.

In this connection I believe we must not overlook the reality that in both the United States and Canada there are at the present time constituencies that fit Hopps' definition of minority status simply by virtue of a combination of geographical location and the virtual extinction of their often long-established economic base and lifestyle. The reasons for the extinction may be relatively direct; for example the collapse of Atlantic fisheries in Canada seems to be the result of decades of over-fishing while the Ministry of Fisheries ignored the scientists' warnings. Others may reflect either changes in demands of industrial standards of cost-efficiency or the introduction of new technology. It will be useful to look at the implications of ethnic-sensitive practice in working with these communities.

These people's identity has for generations been associated with a specific geographical area, and a shared economic base has created that sense of "peoplehood and identification with the group" that Devore and Schlesinger describe. For these minorities in North American society, the apparent hopelessness of recovering their former standard of participation in an economically secure community in their own "homeland" locale is a significant factor in the reality with which they struggle. As social workers in these areas, in attempting to offer help in resolving some of the stress they bring to us, we will also need to take this into account. All too often we have labelled as "apathy" what is in fact a resistance to the pain of having false hopes raised that once more will come to nothing.[3]

Devore and Schlesinger state further that some groups often occupy minority status by virtue of a combination of racism and poverty. In the United States they specifically identify American Indians, Native Alaskans, Mexican Americans, Puerto Ricans, and Asian Americans. In Canada the main groups occupying this status are Native Canadian Indians, and Caribbean and Asian immigrants.

These writers believe that these groups can now be identified in practice as "minorities of color" (Devore and Schlesinger, 1987:513).

For many immigrants, the sense of belonging to an ethnic group can be a source of strength as they begin to deal with how to adapt to the requirements of North American values and way of life. For some, it is of itself a cause of stress because of the perception that as a group—identified either by national origin or skin color or both—there are seemingly insuperable obstacles in the path of their achieving participation in the currently diminishing mainstream of North American life. It also becomes clear to them that this exclusion from opportunity is systemic in origin, sometimes activated by "informally organized" intent, sometimes openly acknowledged. This sense of exclusion, however, is by no means only experienced by immigrant groups. Native North Americans, in both the United States and Canada, have suffered discrimination ever since the establishment of European-style economic and political structures. For lifelong residents of African origin in both countries, discrimination leading to poverty has been a bitter fact of life. In the United States, ever since the abolition of slavery, and in Canada, where historically a haven from slavery was offered, these policies held out an illusory hope of equitable integration into North American social, political, and economic life. They are truly "minorities" in the Hopps definition given above.

One source of stress unique to some members of some ethnic groups comes about, sadly, by reason of their possessing, cultivating, and/or achieving the economic resources that enable them to move into the mainstream of North American life. Financial security, higher education, and/or marketable skills can provide a shift in status away from the main ethnic group. This may result in a measure of rejection by that group and may lead to loss of the psychosocial security provided by the sense of belonging.

The Ethnic Reality Concept

Ethnic-sensitive practice needs to take into account what Devore and Schlesinger call the ethnic reality (1987:514). This is a compound of what a particular group has been socialized to think and feel are the "right"—i.e., customary—ways of ordering community and family life in all their social and economic aspects, patterns of child rearing, and the care of the aged. This encompasses concepts of appropriate gender roles and behaviors in all these interrelationships. There are also the

> psychological bonds of common language, history and sharing of important rituals and celebrations, [and shared habits of feeling and acting that] derive from oppression. (Devore and Schlesinger, 1987:514)

The ethnic reality affects the individual in various ways. Of special significance for social workers may be the client's perception of our role when they seek our service or are directed to us for service. We may be seen as

> a professional helper, appropriately called on to aid in problem-solving, OR as an intruder with no business interfering in intimate matters best kept within the family. (Devore and Schlesinger, 1987:514)

In summary then, in working with these populations, whether in a social service, clinical, group, or community practice context, we shall need to be continually alert to the impact of their ethnic reality. Sometimes the particular difficulties they bring, and their readiness (or difficulty) in accepting the role of client and becoming involved in the helping process, may have specific roots in the fact of their being members of an ethnic group that may be experiencing oppression.

Ethnic-sensitive practice does not require anything "new" in social work principles or strategies. It simply

> . . . involves the adaptation of prevailing social work principles and skills *to take account of the ethnic reality.* (Devore and Schlesinger, 1987:514, emphasis added)

In underlining this these writers cite Norton's definition of ethnic-sensitive practice as being

> . . . a conscious and systematic process of perceiving, understanding and comparing simultaneously the values, attitudes

and behavior of the larger social system with those of the clients' immediate and family system. (1978:3)

Again, this is in essence sound practice with any group of clients. Thus attention to the ethnic reality can be seen as a special facet of the principle of individualization. It requires knowledge of human behavior and of the particular group's history, traditions, values, and mores, and how these may impact upon their use of professional service. Our selective use of models, skills, and methods must take into account the client's ethnic reality as a significant factor in our intervention planning (Devore and Schlesinger, 1987:516).

Implementation of this principle with these, as with all our clients requires self-awareness about our own prejudices. These authors suggest that such self-examination, although uncomfortable, may give insight that can be useful in developing empathy. They also suggest that looking at how our own ethnicity impacts on our self-concept and perception of others–"who am I in the ethnic sense?"–can be helpful in developing greater sensitivity to these clients (Devore and Schlesinger, 1981:83).

ABILITY TO LISTEN AND OBSERVE

Returning now to Biestek's essential worker capacities, we need to understand that what I have called "concerned attention" is the quality that helps the clients begin to share their immediate difficulty and how it feels to them. This is how we begin to learn about who are *these* people and what is *their* trouble.

> The clients want someone to listen to them not just in a friendly way, but in a competent, professional way. . . . Only careful listening to what the clients are saying, and to what they are not saying, can result in our accurately hearing the pertinent material. (adapted from Biestek, 1957:29)

If we are to hear what is being said we must focus on the words used, and, as Biestek also points out, the body language, gestures, facial expressions, seating posture, and mannerisms of the person.

All these may convey feelings about what is or is not being said (1957:29). Our interpretation of what this may reveal also needs to be informed, as has been stated above, by knowledge, understanding, and acceptance of cultural difference. For example, some older North American Indian people were taught that it is disrespectful to look directly in the eyes of an older person or one in a position of authority. An uninformed, white American or Canadian worker could seriously misread this as signalling dishonesty.

In family therapy, frequently the self-selected seating arrangements—who sits beside whom, who takes the chair farthest removed from other family members, and so on—tell us something about the splits and alignments in a family. It will take more than one session for us to verify this as a pattern; we need to establish their trust in our good intentions before it will be appropriate to ask them what they think their choice of seats says about their family relationships. This brings us to Biestek's next requirement in implementing individualization.

Ability to Move at the Client's Pace

> . . . insensitivity to the client's pace can stall the helping process because the client feels that the caseworker is "taking over". . . . Pacing is the guide and test of individualization. (Biestek, 1957:29)

Schlesinger and Devore underline Biestek's point, stating that

> Social workers should demonstrate the capacity to move with each client at a pace and in a direction determined by the client's perception of the problem. . . . understanding that that perception is likely to be affected by the client's ethnicity. (1979:515)

"Taking over" and imposing our own rate of movement upon the client can sometimes be simply a function of our need to be immediately helpful. Devore and Schlesinger's pointed reminder about the possible ethnicity factor in the client's perception of the problem is also important here.

Judgment about pacing is not an easy skill to develop. To be effectively helpful we do need to maintain a certain level of control of the interview's purpose and direction. Maintaining this balance is in part a reflection of our skill in listening and observing. The clients' manifestations of comfort or discomfort–overt or subtle–can be our guide, and experience will gradually enable us to decide when–and when not–to confront the observed difficulty. For example,

> Andrea Dimollo's two children, aged six and four years, are in care of the Child Welfare authority, by a court order, for two months. They had been alone in the family's apartment for two days, while Ms. Dimollo, a single mother, spent the weekend "with a friend." In your sessions, this mother seems to be avoiding the subject of planning for her children's return. As her family worker you may need, at a certain point, to say something like: "I know it's difficult for you to talk about what plans you are able to make for the children's return home to you, but we do need to begin talking about this. We have to work together to have a plan for the court hearing five weeks from now."

The issue of pacing is equally important in working with families. We need to be sensitive to the feelings of each member of the family as they begin to explore with us and with each other how it feels to be present together to talk about what is troubling them. For some families this may be their first experience of coming together for such a purpose. While it is important to observe and identify significant interaction between family members, we need to be careful that we are not hasty in labeling and/or dealing openly with the disclosure of feelings whose expression has quite possibly been taboo in this family's "rules."

The same concerns apply when working with growth-oriented groups. For example, some members will need more time than others to open up their feelings about the purpose of the group; about their concern that the professional leaders carry a "hidden agenda"; about whether the commitment to confidentiality within the group can be taken on faith; and whether it is safe to question this. Helping certain family/group members accept another member's need to move more slowly is an important aspect of the principle of individualization, both as it relates to individual members and to group-building.

Concern about pacing applies equally to work with task-oriented groups and with community projects or organizations. Each group will require our careful attention to the pace of movement that is constructive for them. While helping them to hold to their agreed purpose of each session as a step toward their ultimate objective, we need to be careful that in attempting to "get back on track" we do not appear to belittle their concern about a side issue that they feel requires their time and attention.

Elaboration of these techniques would go beyond the purpose of this volume. They are well covered in helpful books such as Ivey (1988), Shulman (1984), and Cournoyer (1991).

Empathy

The ability to enter into the feelings of people is the fourth quality that Biestek cites as important in the practice implementation of the principle of individualization. It is necessary that we develop our capacity to feel with people and understand and respect that their feelings are individual to them. He identifies warmth as the principal quality in this response (1957:29).

Keefe further clarifies this when he states that

> Although it is possible to understand another person without feeling with him, true empathic skill includes the capacity for an emotional response. (1976:10)

It is this combination of cognitive and feeling responses in the worker that promotes the client's sense of security in exploration and expression of his or her feelings. Rogers illustrates this twofold quality of empathic understanding in his definition:

> . . . the therapist senses accurately the feelings and personal meanings that the client is experiencing and communicates this understanding to the client. (1980:116)

Empathy helps to establish an atmosphere that gives each client a secure feeling that this is a place where "it's safe to be me, *this* me, here and now." For me as a worker, this goes beyond my acceptance of each person's right to his or her own feelings, and assures clients that I am trying to understand and to be truly "with them" in those feelings. I often try to determine whether or not I have accurately heard and understood what they are expressing.

This fulfills two functions. First, it tells my client that I am not assuming that I have heard and understood correctly (Rogers, 1980: 141). Second, it can facilitate the person's exploration and discovery of precisely what is the inner experience they want to communicate. As Rogers states,

> As persons are empathically heard, it becomes possible for them to listen more accurately to the flow of inner experiencings. (1980:116)

The quality of warmth–of caring–is an essential ingredient in empathy (Biestek, 1957:29). Rogers calls this "unconditional positive regard" (1980:116). It is this quality that will communicate the feeling of safety, and convey that we are really "with" this person and trying our best to understand how they feel.[4]

The unconditional quality of the worker's caring requires attention to the principles of self-awareness and acceptance. We need to acknowledge–inwardly–when the client's feelings touch us, arousing an old fear, perhaps, or strong disapproval. We shall need to recognize that the fear and disapproval originate in us and do not belong in the client's here and now; we also need to remind ourselves of this person's right to his or her own feelings, and to reassure ourselves that those feelings cannot in any way harm or overwhelm us.

In this way we can provide the climate in which the client feels safe to explore events, feelings, and meanings that are fearful for them. Rogers beautifully expresses this process as including

> . . . communicating your sensings of the person's world as you look with fresh and unfrightened eyes at elements of which he

or she is fearful. . . . *You are a confident companion to the person in his or her inner world.* (1980:142, emphasis added)

Ability to Keep Perspective

This is the sixth quality Biestek identifies as necessary in the implementation of the principle of individualization. It requires that we control our emotional involvement and direct our focus to the client's total situation. In this way we can constantly maintain a perspective that

> helps [us] to see the feelings as they are related to the objective situation and the individual as he is related to his family and social situation. (Biestek, 1957:30)

Maintaining perspective is easier when we keep in mind the interrelationship of the clients with their political, economic, familial, and community environment (Schlesinger and Devore, 1979: 513). This approach is also in keeping with the systems model of practice that Bartlett's definition, cited earlier, makes clear. She states, in part:

> Thus person and situation, people and environment are encompassed in a single concept, which requires that they be constantly reviewed together. (Bartlett, 1970:104)

We need to keep in mind that the individuality of each client, or group of clients, is a factor in this composite. In some instances the presenting difficulty may directly reflect discrepancies between "the [person's, family's, group's, or organization's] coping activities and the demands of their environment" (Bartlett, 1970:104). Perspective is also facilitated when we do not lose sight of individual client strengths.

This interconnectedness is of course also a factor to be considered when dealing with the members of a formed group. For example, a group of women shoplifters on probation have not only been defined as lawbreakers by the Court, representing society, but may include some who are estranged from their family, either because of their offense, or due to some longer-standing dissension. The crime itself, in some instances, may be in part a response to experiences of communal and/or familial rejection. It may also have been–and may still be–a source of approval, even recognition, from a peer group in which they have a strong–perhaps their only–sense of belonging.

A group of physically abusive parents, whose children are in care of the child welfare system, must usually live daily with the overt and/or subtle disapproval of neighbors, and in some cases of their extended families also. They have also experienced the explicit condemnation, via court proceedings, of the larger community.

At the community practice level, the following example will show the importance of maintaining this overall perspective in responding to the request for service.

A group of residents in a city neighborhood of low-cost, run-down rooming houses are young and middle-aged men and women, discharged from psychiatric hospital care, receiving various forms of social assistance. They are led by three vocal and active young people–two men and one woman–who plan to take action to obtain permission (and some basic funding) from the city to establish a cooperative gardening project on part of a vacant lot in their neighborhood. The leaders had found that the gardening they did while in the hospital was very rewarding, and they believe such a project will revive the spirits of their coresidents. They also think they might sell the flowers and perhaps vegetables on a communal basis. They have already begun a clean-up job on the vacant lot to show their good faith as they approach the authorities. They are seeking advice and help from their social assistance and disability pension workers on how to approach local government officials.

As their workers, it will be important that we keep in mind the overall situation of these people. First, these people experience the stigma of mental illness and unemployment on a daily basis (they may be labeled as "welfare bums"). These attitudes are likely pervasive among their landlords and the householders and store keepers in the same area. They will certainly be encountered in meetings with municipal officials as we help these clients advocate for their neighborhood project. We shall need to help them hold on to their–and one would hope our– vision of what this project could mean and achieve for them in terms of enhanced feelings of self-worth and interest in life. But they–and we–will need to take into account (and strategize to overcome) the likely reality of a general public perception that this is just a "hare-brained scheme of a bunch of crazies." The creative imagination of the activists may possibly be threatened by some degree of apathy or even defeatism from some of their more despondent coresidents. As their social workers, we need to guard against being infected by these negative attitudes, while we also must not minimize the realistic difficulties with which the project will have to contend.

Flexibility

Biestek's list of thoughtfulness in details, privacy in interviews, care in keeping appointments, etc. (1957:30-32), as means of individualizing, has mainly been dealt with in the chapter "Respect for Human Worth and Dignity." His suggestion of the need for flexibility, however, highlights an important practical expression of individualization.

As we learn and understand more about our clients, Biestek says, we need to be ready to modify the objectives, as well as the methods, of our interventions. Changes in their life situation and within the persons themselves may alter their view of what they need and want to work toward. Biestek says it is important that we develop the judgment, objectivity, and skill to adapt goals and methods to take such changes into account, and that this "is a specific way of individualizing the client" (1957:32).

Individualization is one of the cardinal principles of professional social work. Its implementation in practice can make the crucial difference between a truly professional, personalized kind of help and a technically competent but uninvolved "processing" of troubled persons. The pain and struggles of different people may look the same to us, but we must never assume that they fit a familiar mold and will respond to "what works in such cases." To be truly helpful we must keep a central truth in the forefront of all our thinking and our direct intervention with clients; this is that each person, each family, and each group or organization of persons, experiences the reality of their life situation in ways that are unique to who they are.

SUMMARY OF MAIN POINTS

1. Individualization is based on the right of human beings to be treated as *this* human being, not just *a* human being.
2. Individualization requires some specific capacities in the worker for its implementation:
   (a) Freedom from bias and prejudice: this involves self-awareness in facing and identifying our prejudices and biases for what they are; it also requires controlled emotional involvement and a nonjudgmental attitude.
   (b) Knowledge of human behavior and of theories of practice: this includes knowledge of the various socioeconomic, ethnic, and religious cultures of the community where we work, and understanding the concept of "ethnic reality."
   (c) The skills of listening and observing: these are integral to the implementation of this principle.
   (d) The ability to move at the clients' pace: we need to give them the time they need to work toward the agreed-upon goals of change; this may require that we curb our need to be immediately helpful, but in some cases time constraints are a reality for us and the clients.
   (e) The ability to enter into people's feelings, i.e., empathy: this will involve self-awareness, warmth, unconditional positive regard, and a nonjudgmental acceptance of each person's right to be him/herself and to their own feelings.
   (f) The ability to keep perspective: this involves our continued attention to the individual's, group's, or organization's total environmental system as a part of the reality within which they are individually struggling.
   (g) Flexibility in our work with clients: this may mean being ready to modify both our goals and our methods of intervention as our clients redefine their need or desire for change.

NOTES

1. Systems theory has become so much a part of our professional knowledge base that we may forget that it came to us initially from the physical sciences via von Bertalanffy, a theoretical biologist (Berrien, 1968:5).

2. Sir William Osler, a noted Canadian physician, told his students, "Ask not what disease the person has, ask what person the disease has."

3. Although not "minorities" within the definition being used here, *many* of these factors will be present in work with the increasing numbers of persons whose well-established economic security and lifestyle has collapsed due to technological displacement at their workplace.

4. It is all too easy to say, "I know how you feel." I do not believe we can ever "know" this, and it is certainly presumptuous to say so unless we confirm a client's feelings by asking, "Are you saying that. . . ?"

REFERENCES

Bartlett, Harriet M. (1970). *The Common Base of Social Work Practice.* Washington, DC: National Association of Social Workers.

Berrien, F. Kenneth. (1968). *General and Social Systems.* New Brunswick, NJ: Rutgers University Press.

Biestek, Felix P. (1957). *The Casework Relationship.* Chicago, IL: Loyola University Press.

Cournoyer, Barry. (1991). *Social Work Skills Workbook.* Belmont, CA: Wadsworth Publishing.

Devore, Wynetta and Elfrieda Schlesinger. (1987). "Ethnic Sensitive Practice." *Encyclopedia of Social Work,* 18th edition. Volume 1: 512-516.

———— (1981). *Ethnic Sensitive Social Work Practice, First Edition.* St. Louis, MO: C.V. Mosby Co.

Erikson, Erik. (1950). *Childhood and Society.* New York: W.W. Norton & Company.

———— (1980). *Identity and the Life Cycle.* New York: W.W. Norton & Company.

Garrett, Annette. (1942). *Interviewing: Its Principles and Methods.* New York: Family Welfare Association of America.

Gordon, Milton M. (1964). *Assimilation in American Life.* New York: Oxford University Press. Cited in Devore and Schlesinger. (1987). "Ethnic Sensitive Practice." *Encyclopedia of Social Work,* 18th edition. Volume 1: 513.

Hopps, June Gary. (1983-1984). "Minorities: People of Color." *Supplement to the Encyclopedia of Social Work,* 17th Edition. Silver Spring, MD: 76-83.

Ivey, Allen E. (1988). *Intentional Interviewing and Counseling, Second Edition.* Pacific Grove, CA: Brooks/Cole.

Keefe, Thomas. (1976). "Empathy: The Critical Skill." *Social Work,* 21(1):10-14.

Norton, Dolores G. (1978). *The Dual Perspective: Inclusion of Ethnic Minority Content in the Social Work Curriculum*. New York: Council of Social Work Education.

Osler, William. cited in Sacks, Oliver. (1995). *An Anthropologist on Mars*. Toronto, Canada: Alfred A. Knopf.

Rogers, Carl. (1980). *A Way of Being*. Boston: Houghton Mifflin Company, pp. 113-134, 137-161.

Schlesinger, Elfrieda and Wynetta Devore. (1979). "Social Workers View Ethnic Minority Teaching." *Journal of Social Work Education*, (15)3:20-27.

Shulman, L. (1984). *The Skills of Helping People and Groups*. Chicago, IL: F.E. Peacock.

OTHER USEFUL READING

For Canadian students, a valuable resource about work with Cree and Ojibway Native groups in Northern Canada is:

Ross, Rupert. (1992). *Dancing with a Ghost: Exploring Indian Reality*. Markham, ON, Canada: Octopus Publishing.

Chapter 10

Purposeful Expression of Feelings:
A Necessary Element
in Effective Helping

This principle plays a key role in helping people to develop or recover healthy psychosocial functioning. In earlier chapters attention was paid to the worker's need for self-awareness about his or her own comfort with–or anxiety about–the client's expression of feelings. This chapter will focus on the specific therapeutic value of the expression of feelings as an integral part of the helping process. Some method suggestions are included.

Implementation of this principle requires that

> workers recognize their clients' need to express their feelings freely, including their negative feelings, and that clients can do this where they know that they are accepted and treated as an individual. The worker listens purposefully, neither discouraging nor condemning the expression of feelings, and at times actively stimulating and encouraging them as a part of the helping process. (adapted from Biestek, 1957:35)

In helping clients we must always take into account how they feel, as well as what they think about their situation. The troubled person's feelings are integral to his or her perception of the difficulty, and are involved in any ideas he or she may have about possible solutions.

Indeed, the feelings may be the most difficult part of the problem (Biestek, 1957:37).

Because we believe in the therapeutic value of opening the self to what has been hidden, we must attempt to help clients achieve a level of trust with us that frees them to share both thoughts and feelings. This may include their negative feelings about needing our help, about the limitations of agency service relative to their felt needs, and perhaps about us as helpers. Some clients may express these feelings quite early in the contact, depending upon their degree of self-confidence and their degree of trust that this will not result in our rejecting their request for help. Others may conceal their negative feelings about these things, more or less effectively, until either they feel safe in expressing them, or we, sensing that they need to express them, encourage them to do so.

We have discussed earlier the importance of accepting the feelings of our clients without shock, disapproval, or inner anxiety that may stem from unresolved issues in our own lives. Here I want to emphasize our need to be acutely tuned in to what the client may be feeling, and to what they are trying—or trying not—to express; we need to reassure them that it will be safe to express it with us.

THE THERAPEUTIC PURPOSE
OF EXPRESSING FEELINGS

Biestek states that the expression of feelings can accomplish four purposes (Biestek 1957:37-38). Each will be discussed and some examples will be given to illustrate them in action.

The Relief of Pressures and Tensions, to Free the Client for Positive, Constructive Action

Clients are frequently blocked from taking constructive action to resolve or relieve the stress of their problem situation by unacknowledged feelings that freeze their ability to act.

Dennis K. came to the college counseling service in late February, on recommendation of one of his professors and the dean of the small college residence where he was living. Dennis was an exceptionally bright student, but his marks had gone down badly since Christmas. His relationships with his roommate and with others in residence had deteriorated since late November and were creating problems for him and for the general management of the residence.

Initially Dennis appeared very concerned about his low marks, saying that lately he could not concentrate and would "go for a drink with anyone" rather than hit the books. When Marvin, the counselor, asked about the fighting and difficulties in residence, Dennis said he felt he had discovered that his roommates were "just not his type," and this made it hard, as he knew he must stick it out until the end of the year.

At the second interview Marvin explored Dennis' family background. His mother died of cancer when he was four years old. He was the youngest of three children, and his sisters were eight and eleven years old at the time. Their father had held things together by moving in with his married sister. Their aunt and uncle had no children of their own and were very kind, warmly welcoming the family. Their father urged them to be "brave" and not cry for mother, because Auntie was so good to them. All the children became close with their aunt, especially Dennis.

This arrangement was maintained until Dennis was seven years old, at which time his father remarried and established a home with his new wife and the children in a city some distance from where they had previously lived. Mr. K felt that he needed to establish his wife's position as the children's stepmother and purposely did not arrange for regular, let alone frequent, meetings with their aunt and uncle. All the children got along well with their stepmother, who was very good to them.

Dennis was fifteen when his stepmother was killed in a car accident. His father, who was driving the car, was injured, but not seriously, and he recovered. He and the two girls, both still living at home, maintained the family home thereafter. Mr. K was very depressed for several months, but he recovered and things went on fairly well.

Dennis, now nineteen, was in his first year at college—his first year away from home. His eldest sister married last year, and his next sister had just graduated with a degree in nursing and was planning to live independently in a few months.

During the previous summer his father had begun dating another woman, and at Thanksgiving he told the family that he and Lauranne were going to get married.

At first Dennis had liked Lauranne very much, and could see that she thought a lot of his father. She was warm and friendly to him and the girls. When his father told the family that he and Lauranne intended to marry and move to a new house, Dennis said he began to see that she "just wasn't right for Dad." He began to be very critical of everything about her, sometimes even to her face. Marvin gathered that at Christmas Dennis had made things so unpleasant for himself and everyone else that his father had suggested that he start looking for a summer job that would enable him to live elsewhere.

Exploring this history with Dennis, Marvin was struck by the unemotional way he talked about the various losses. Marvin suggested that these losses must have been painful for him. Dennis said in a matter-of-fact way that yes, it was sad at the time, but "that was all in the past." Exploring this further, Marvin learned that when their mother died, their aunt would not allow them to cry about it, because seeing them cry would "upset their dad." When they left his aunt and uncle, Dennis remembered that he had missed his aunt at first, but his father had said it was "unkind" to their stepmother if they seemed to pine for their aunt. Their stepmother was good to them and they all got along well. When Dennis's stepmother died, the doctor had advised (and the girls had agreed) that, because of their father's depression, "We must be strong for Dad's sake."

When Marvin asked about Lauranne, Dennis set his jaw in a defiant way and said he could see she was "just after Dad's money." For Thanksgiving, his father and the girls had cooked a great turkey dinner. Lauranne had turned up "just in time to eat," and brought homemade cranberry sauce, "of all things." Marvin said, "That made you angry?" Dennis said it did. Marvin asked if the cranberry sauce was good. Dennis shrugged and said it was "nothing special."

Marvin said gently, "Sounds like you think she can't do anything right?" Dennis sneered and tried to laugh, but he choked and began to cry. Marvin said he had a right to cry, and moved his chair a little closer to Dennis's.

This proved to be the breakthrough that Dennis needed: to admit his fear that if he got close to Lauranne she would leave him as the other mother figures in his life had. As he told Marvin about this, he began to recognize and accept that this fear and its accompanying anger were also at the root of his problems with his grades and his relationships on campus.

Discussion

> Give sorrow words. The grief that does not speak, whispers the o'er-fraught heart, and bids it break. (Shakespeare, *Macbeth*)

This client had never been allowed to express his grief at the loss of three mother figures, beginning with the loss of his birth mother at age four. In each instance the expression of feeling was disapproved of on the grounds of its hurting someone else's feelings. No one had heard the inner child's cry: "What about *my* feelings?" Dennis presented himself with the situational problems of his college grades and relationships with other students. The worker did not focus exclusively on this but rather moved to examine Dennis's many losses. His reaction to Lauranne was clearly the key. His anger, expressed at home by sarcastic criticism of Lauranne and at college by being quarrelsome and disrespectful to everybody, was the clue. The worker considered the possibility that Dennis may have been "angry on the outside, frightened on the inside; frightened on the outside, angry on the inside."[1]

The worker's insight freed Dennis to express feelings that had been bottled up from his early childhood. This allowed him to move out of the position in which he was "stuck," feeling there was nothing he could do about his current problems and he must "stick it out till the end of term." Acknowledging the real origin of his anger and unhappiness, Dennis was able to begin to accept his pent-up grief as valid. He was able to look at his low grades and fighting in the residence and see that these self-defeating behaviors were totally ineffective ways of dealing with his fear of further loss. The release of his feelings freed Dennis "for positive, constructive action" (Biestek, 1957:38).

This is what Greenberg and Safran call

> emotional restructuring, that is, evoking the [emotional] network underlying problematic responses in order to re-structure the network. (1989:23-24)

It may seem like a very small point that the worker moved his chair closer to this young man while he cried, but it served as a nonintrusive but definite way of showing Dennis that the worker was "with" him at that crucial emotional point.

Expressed Feelings Give a Deeper Understanding of the Significance the Client Attaches to Certain Facets of the Problem

The following case illustrates this aspect of the therapeutic purpose.

> A group of five overweight women, ages thirty-five to forty-five, were meeting at an eating disorders clinic to learn about weight control. None of the women were suffering from a specific eating disorder, but all were "yo-yo dieters" who felt their weight caused difficulties for them in various areas of their lives. They wanted to learn how to reduce and control their weight in a lasting way.
>
> Kate and Nathalie, the two staff members, made it clear that the main purpose of the group was educational. They would be talking about nutrition, eating patterns, types of favored foods, the timing of meals and snacks, the link between overeating and/or certain foods with the aftermath of certain events, the avoidance of "miracle" and other diets, and so on. But they also emphasized that how the group members *felt* about food and what their overeating did to them would also be discussed, but only when the group members felt comfortable enough to raise those issues.
>
> As the group process developed, some of the women began to talk about their feelings, and about the general societal perception that fat people were not as good as other people. Marg cried as she said that she decided to join the group when she learned that her eight-year-old son had not told her about the

school field day. The last time she was at a school event, some kids had teased him about his "big fat mom."

Nathalie reminded the women that they would need to look at weight loss and weight control as something they were doing for themselves, not because of what others thought. She quoted a TV commercial for a cosmetic that concluded with a woman saying, "And I'm *worth it*!"

Louellen started to cry. The woman next to her put her arm round her shoulder, and Louellen poured out her feeling that she was simply not worth anything at all. She was the youngest and the third girl in her family, ten years younger than her next sister. Their father operated a business founded by his grandfather. She had never felt "wanted" by either of her parents, and when she was about seven her paternal grandmother had told her "we really didn't need another girl." When Louellen had cried about this, her grandmother ridiculed her for being "sensitive," and said it was "a joke."

Both her older sisters had done well in school, academically and in sports, whereas Louellen had found school a struggle. She was "chubby" as a child, and started to get overweight in her teens. She knew she had overeaten ever since she could remember, and she believed her weight had made her unpopular at school with girls as well as boys. She had never married, but when she was twenty years old she had had a child. ("A one-night stand, like a whore, but I didn't get paid!") The father of the child had left town as soon as she told him she was pregnant. She had given the baby up for adoption.

The picture that emerged from Louellen's story was of a woman who—possibly from birth onwards—had never received the kind of nurturing acceptance that children need to develop a healthy sense of self-worth. "I hate myself," she said at one point.

After this meeting, Kate asked Louellen to stay behind. She suggested that some individual counseling, along with attendance at the group, might help her with her profound lack of self-worth. Clearly the pattern she had described of losing weight and regaining it was closely linked to her deep feeling that she did not *deserve* to look nice, to be attractive, to make the most of her appearance.

Louellen agreed and was linked up with one of the therapists on the clinic staff. She continued going to the group meetings, and through developing better feelings about her own self-worth she made good use of the suggested changes in eating patterns and lifestyle on which the group work focused.

Discussion

Weight problems are frequently associated with emotional factors of varying kinds and degrees, such as low self-esteem and depression. North American culture penalizes obesity, especially in women, associating it with a negative judgement about people's worth, and this attitude is readily absorbed by many overweight people.

Although the main purpose of the group was educational, it was made clear to the members from the outset that their feelings were to be included in the group's deliberations. This opened the way for participants to express the feelings they attached to their difficulty in attaining and maintaining a weight that was satisfactory to them as individuals.

For Louellen it was clear that her weight problem was only one manifestation of a deep-seated lack of self-worth. No amount of "education" about changing eating patterns and lifestyle would have any effect for this woman unless her feelings of low self-worth were addressed at the same time. The opportunity offered by the workers allowed Louellen to express her lack of self-esteem.

Kate picked up on this. She understood the depth of Louellen's feelings and that they were going to obstruct her use of the main content of the group's program. This led to the development of an effective helping process for this young woman to change her life in positive ways.

Listening to and Accepting the Expression of Feelings Is a Form of Psychological Support

We need to remember that even where they have been aware of their own strong feelings, many of our clients have hidden from

others their real feelings about certain events, relationships, or experiences. When they feel fully accepted and can trust our concern for
them as genuine, they will begin to open up to us. The psychological
purpose of the expression of feelings is important in that a burden is
less onerous when it is shared (Biestek, 1957:38).

> Jane had told me a very painful story of a series of impulsive
> choices that had turned out to be disastrous moves for herself
> and her children. These led to a situation of being alone with
> the children, living on social assistance in substandard hous-
> ing. Her family were totally unsympathetic, rubbing it in that
> her situation was her "own fault." She tried not to cry in front
> of her children, who were preschoolers, because she knew it
> upset them. Crying alone at night made her recognize her
> loneliness and the reasons for it, which she knew were in fact
> largely "her own fault."
> As she wept, she told me, "It's so good to sit here and cry."
> She felt supported by my acceptance of her right to cry, and by
> my lack of any blame-placing.

We must not underrate the importance of this kind of support. We
all need someone to be truly *with* us when we are in trouble, and it is
part of our professional responsibility to be fully there for each
client when they need that. Our silence, and perhaps our small,
thoughtful gestures, can reassure them that we are with them in their
pain.[2]

Some people have difficulty in letting go and expressing their
feelings, and we need to accept that. We may "know" that it would
help them to let go and cry, but if they have never learned to trust
anyone that far, all we can do is behave in ways that will convey our
genuine caring and concern. As a client of mine was telling me
about a desperately troubled childhood, she kept forcefully knuck-
ling away tears from her cheeks. I suggested that she might feel
better if she "let go and cry about this."

She told me, "You don't understand, if you let people know how
much you hurt, they'll use it against you." My immediate inner
reaction was: "But I'm not like that!" but I knew that telling her this
was futile. She needed time to experience for herself that I was
trustworthy.

In this instance one could ask if it was my need for her to cry, or hers, that I was trying to meet? Knowing that crying could relieve her, I came close to pushing her to "do what I thought best" for her. My acceptance of her inability to let go is an example of offering psychological support for this person's individuality. We need to recognize that expression of feelings is only purposeful when the client is ready. As noted earlier, this readiness can be verified with such comments as "I should think that must have hurt you a lot," or "Some people would find that pretty scary."

Where the Client's Negative Feelings Are Part of the Problem, Purposeful Expression Brings Them Out into the Open so That Something Can Be Done About Them

The Louellen case discussed above is one example of the value of the expression of negative feelings–in her case these feelings were directed toward herself–as a step toward resolving the client's problem. Negative feelings toward others can of course also be an important factor in the difficulties that clients bring to us.

Suppressed anger can effectively obstruct movement toward making constructive change. It can interfere with healthy growth, and prevent the formation of healthy and productive relationships in the family and in work situations. Speaking specifically of anger, DeFoore suggests that

> Feelings are just like vegetables. . . . The longer we leave our feelings inside without expressing them, the more unpleasant they become. . . . They get hot and generate energy, which has to come out one way or another. (1991:20-21)

Adult children of abusive parents, adult survivors of sexual abuse, and adult children of alcoholics can all be struggling with an inner anger that for different reasons they have never allowed themselves to express. DeFoore lists some of the reasons why we may learn in childhood to bury anger. Parents who never express anger or raise their voices, give their children a clear message that "we don't act that way here." They may also imply: "If you act ugly we won't love you." Child victims of sexual and physical abuse usually feel blameworthy, partly if not wholly, which can lead them to think: "I have no right to be angry."

Lastly a child may be punished severely by parents for expressing anger, the message being again that anger is bad and we will not be loved if we get angry. In other families no emotions of any kind are expressed, giving the message that all feelings are bad (DeFoore, 1991:11-12). The repression of anger may also be culturally influenced. In Western society we are at present uncertain as to whether we still believe that controlling anger plays a role in maintaining social order.[3]

Many of us in practice have seen the anxious clinging of some clients to a dream picture of parents who "loved us deep down" yet were consistently cold and distant with their children, or were so stern and disapproving of all misdemeanors that their children grew up to believe that unless they were perfect, they were of no worth at all. I asked one client how he knew his parents loved him. He replied, "We were always well-dressed, we had good meals, and were sent to school." I found this a very chilling description of minimal parental care. The clinging to what I have called the "dream picture" is a way of escaping the childhood verdict of "I am unlovable," but it is also a way of keeping the unexpressed anger at bay.

Helping some clients reach the point of acknowledging their anger may be a fairly long process, but an explicit reassurance that they have a right to be angry is helpful. The next step, expressing that anger, can have dramatic results in terms of release from the prison of anxiety and passivity. DeFoore's clinic is specially set up for the physical expression of anger in a safe way, with pounding fists on a pillow, but he describes specific safeguards that not every service can provide (1991:106-112).

It is very helpful to many clients to write the kind of letter to the abusive parent that they have no intention of mailing. They can say what has never been said in a safe way, and they can be reassured that such letters can be destroyed in the office after reading.

Doug came to the family counseling center requesting help with working out a troubled relationship with his parents. His father had recently been diagnosed with terminal cancer at an advanced stage. Doug wanted to be there for his mother during this difficult time, but his feelings from the past about his father prevented him from doing this.

Doug said he was still bitter about his father's treatment of him and his sister, which did indeed sound both psychologically and physically cruel. After they left home he and his sister had virtually cut themselves off from their parents, visiting them two or three times a year on special occasions. These visits were strained because their father disagreed with almost anything they said, and was sarcastic about their chosen work, their relatively low incomes, and their modest living circumstances. Doug was twenty-six, and after a couple of false starts in other lines of work he had taken an extensive computer course. For the past six months he had been very happily working with a local firm that sold and serviced computers. He felt confident, and had been told by his superiors that he had good prospects there. His older sister had recently married and she and her husband, both working outside the home, were saving to buy a house.

Since his father's illness Doug had begun to realize that his parents were in fact very lonely people. His father's personality had prevented them from making any real friends, either at work or since retirement.

Pauline, Doug's worker, suggested that he write a letter to his father–a letter he had no intention of mailing–telling his father just how he felt about his treatment of the children, including things he especially remembered feeling bad about. Doug said he would try to do that. He was to bring the letter to the next interview, and they would read it together and destroy it in the office, if that's what Doug wanted.

When Doug offered her the letter he had written he apologized to Pauline, an older woman, for some of the language he had used. Pauline reassured him again that he had a right to be angry and to express it however it came out. It would not shock her. His pen had almost gone through the paper in places as he began to let out his pent-up rage. Doug cried several times as he read the letter out loud, but he said it was extraordinary how relieved he felt after "getting all that out in the open." The fact that it felt so "safe" to do this had helped him; he knew it was not going to hurt his dad, or his mother. He asked Pauline to keep the letter in his file, as he "might want to look it over again."

As they worked together further, Pauline asked about what his mother had done when his dad was being so cruel. Doug said his mother had always been "just Dad's shadow," completely subservient and never expressing any needs of her own. He "guessed she had been a good mother," but she had never stood up for the children or tried to get their father to be kinder to them.

In talking about this, Doug began to realize that, although he had felt sorry for his mother since he left home, lately he had begun to see her more clearly in her self-imposed victim role, and he realized that he felt some bottled-up anger against her. "She could at least have comforted us sometimes," he said, with tears in his eyes. Pauline suggested he write a letter to her. He seemed very uncertain about this and Pauline asked what was making it hard for him. Doug replied that he wondered if he had the right to be angry with her, knowing as he did now that she had been just as afraid of his Dad as he and his sister were.

Pauline said he had the right to feel angry with her, for the little boy he once was. Doug asked if she meant it was okay to "kind of take his side against her?" and Pauline said that for his present purpose it definitely was.

At the next appointment, Doug said that in thinking about this letter, he had remembered some good "motherly" things about his mother when he was very small, and this had helped him. He guessed that while the children were really young their dad had not taken much interest in them and so his mother had been more free to be "motherly." He had remembered that when he was about six he had badly scraped his knee; his mother was comforting him and his dad "yelled that she was making a sissy crybaby of me." Doug believed she became afraid of his father's anger and had to stop being "motherly." In the letter he was able to express some of his anger about his mother not standing up to his father, and he cried as he read out loud: "Couldn't you see how small we felt compared to HIM?"

At the next interview they reviewed what these exercises (and talking about them) had done for Doug. He said that besides a great release of feelings, he felt "grown-up" in a new way with his parents, and a recent visit had been much less stressful. He said that at one point during the visit his father's sarcasm had triggered the old feelings, but he had said to himself, "No, he's a poor, sick old man and I'm grown up now." This had helped him not to take it personally, as he would have before. As Doug stood up, ready to leave, Pauline took the letters out of the file and asked Doug what he would like to do with them. Doug made a dismissive gesture toward the wastebasket. "Just pitch them," he said.[4]

Discussion

This client had good insight into his difficulties, and was motivated by his father's terminal illness to work out a relationship with his parents that would allow him to be with them both through a difficult time. Writing the letters allowed him to express, in complete safety, negative feelings from the past that were the main part of the problem in his relationship with his parents. This method of expressing such feelings helped him to begin relating to his parents—especially to his father—as an adult son, relieved of the emotional load of childhood pain he had been carrying.

Not all clients are as ready to express their feelings as Doug. As noted earlier, we must not "push" those who are less ready, but ensure that we do offer them enough stimulus for expression of feelings. There is a danger that we may underestimate these clients' ego strength and rush in to express their feelings for them. This can block them from the work of expressing feelings that, although painful, may be a necessary part of the helping process (Biestek, 1957:44).

PURPOSEFUL LIMITATIONS

There are, of course, limits to the expression of feelings, and some of these will now be considered.

Agency Function and Structures

We need to limit the expression of feelings to "those with which the agency's service is designed to deal" (Biestek, 1957:39). Greenberg and Safran (1989) and DeFoore (1991) describe techniques that may be used to intensify emotional awareness, so that clients can give physical expression to a remembered image of a traumatic experience, in order to express the feelings that were aroused at the time. Greenberg and Safran stress, however, that such techniques should only be used by "therapists comfortable with and knowledgeable about working with emotion" (1989:26).

Caseload size, perhaps increasingly a major factor today, may limit the frequency of contact, and thus may impose restriction on our facilitating expression of feelings. We must recognize that clients encouraged to reveal very deep feelings may need more frequent interviews, over a certain period of time, than our caseloads permit. The availability of psychiatric consultation must also be taken into account in some cases, depending on the nature of the feelings, the worker's capabilities, and the assessment of the client's ego strength or fragility (Biestek, 1957:45).

Risk of Premature Expression of Deep Feelings

We also need to be careful about the risks inherent in the premature venting of deep feelings. Sometimes it can arouse in the client guilty feelings and regret. It can also bring about a feeling of having been "tricked" into revealing more than the client was ready to reveal. Either can result in "purposeless hostility toward the worker" (Biestek, 1957:40).

It is particularly important that Intake workers guard against this. Sharing deep feelings, and finding that these are accepted by the worker, deepens the relationship. This can make the transfer to the ongoing worker more difficult (Biestek, 1957:40).

Risk of Perpetuating Dependency

The troubled client needs and benefits from a certain level of dependency in the helping relationship. We need to see this as necessary and temporary. If we are oversupportive psychologically, we risk preventing precisely the kind of personal growth that needs to be the shared objective of the helping process. Such oversupport, or overprotectiveness, can arise from our own need to be needed.

Again, the crucial question is: "Whose need is being met here?" We need to remember that "success" is when our clients do not need us any more.

THE EXPRESSION OF FEELINGS AS AN AID IN STUDY, ASSESSMENT, AND INTERVENTION PLANNING

If clients are allowed to tell their story in their own words and to talk about how they feel, we are able to gain an increasingly clear picture of the pertinent reality of the situation with which they are struggling. We gain a picture of these persons' strengths and areas of difficulty, and valuable clues as to which aspects of the problem they could most comfortably and practically address in beginning the work of desired change. As some of the examples above have shown, the expression of feelings helps clients begin to see their problems more clearly, and to begin looking at what action they might take to resolve them.

If change is to be of real and lasting value, it is essential that clients involve themselves in the process. How they feel about change is an integral part of the reality of the helping process and must be taken into account in the intervention plan (Biestek, 1957:47).

SUMMARY OF MAIN POINTS

1. The purposeful expression of feelings is an important factor in the helping relationship, and has a number of specific purposes in the therapeutic endeavor.
2. Workers must strive to create an atmosphere of trust and acceptance, such that clients feel safe in expressing all kinds of feelings, some of which they may not previously have allowed into their awareness.
3. Unacknowledged feelings can sometimes mask the real nature of the problem for the client and thus block constructive action toward its resolution.

4. The expression of feelings can help clients and workers understand how much significance is attached to particular aspects of the problem.
5. Our readiness to listen to the expression of feelings, without judging, gives clients psychological support and thus deepens the relationship.
6. The expression of feelings is only purposeful when the client is ready. We need to keep a balance between facilitating but not pushing the clients' expression of feelings.
7. Expressing negative feelings brings them out in the open so that something can be done about them. Clients need to know that we are not shocked or upset if they express negative feelings about shortcomings they see in us as workers, or in the service that is being offered.
8. Agency function will limit the appropriateness of expression of feelings in some instances.
9. Intake workers need to be careful that they do not allow too much expression of deep feelings, since this may make it more difficult for clients to transfer to the ongoing worker.
10. We need to keep the therapeutic purpose at the center of our attention, and ensure that we do not encourage the expression of feelings for its own sake. This can lead us to encourage dependency beyond what is needed and therapeutic for our clients.
11. The expression of feelings can be an important aid in study, assessment, and intervention planning.

NOTES

1. While this should not be applied universally as a "rule of thumb," it is often worth testing where history suggests its relevance. If it does not make sense to the client, either because it does not apply, or because they are not ready to deal with it, they will simply reject it, and we let it go.

2. This, as noted earlier, is part of what is truly professional in social work: the offering to our clients that "fullness of humanity" of which Biestek speaks (1957:131).

3. Physical expressions of rage in sports are generally tolerated now, although they were relatively unheard of in the past.

4. A client of mine made a private ritual burning of her letters on the barbecue. With a very expressive gesture she told me, "It all just went up in smoke."

REFERENCES

Biestek, Felix P. (1957). *The Casework Relationship*. Chicago, IL: Loyola University Press.

DeFoore, Bill. (1991). *Anger: Deal with It, Heal with It, Stop It From Killing You*. Deerfield Beach, FL: Health Communications Inc.

Greenberg, Leslie S. and Jeremy D. Safran. (1989). "Emotion in Psychotherapy." *The American Psychologist*, 44(1):19-29.

Shakespeare, William. (circa 1600). "Macbeth," IV, iii. In *William Shakespeare: The Complete Works*. Peter Alexander, ed. London and Glasgow: Collins, 1951, p. 1021.

Chapter 11

Self-Determination:
A Right of All Clients

Self-determination has been a central principle of professional social work practice since the 1930s. Its significance stemmed initially from observation that help of any kind was more effective if the client participated in the helping process. From this evolved a philosophical conviction that the client had a natural right to make his or her own choices and decisions (Biestek, 1957:101-103).

According to Biestek, this right is

   (i) a necessary, fundamental right of the client flowing from his essential dignity as a human being;

  (ii) a necessary fundamental right of all individuals in a democratic society;

 (iii) necessary for the effectiveness of casework [and all social work] service and treatment; and

 (iv) an essential principle in casework [social work] philosophy. (1957:104)

Biestek defines the principle as follows:

the practical recognition of the right and need of clients to freedom in making their own choices and decisions in the [social work] process, and that [social workers] have a corresponding duty to

• respect that right,
• recognize that need,

- stimulate and help to activate that potential for self-direction by helping the client to see and use the available and appropriate resources of the community and his own personality.

The client's right to self-determination, however, is limited by

- the client's capacity for positive and constructive decision-making;
- the framework of the civil and moral law; and
- the function of the agency. (1957:103)

Each of these limitations has practice implications and will be discussed in some detail later in this chapter.

OBLIGATIONS UNDER THE CODE OF ETHICS

The NASW Code of Ethics (1993) also recognizes that the right to self-determination must be qualified in some degree, but emphasizes that "the social worker should make every effort to foster maximum self-determination on the part of clients" (II, G:6). Three consequent obligations are specified:

1. When the social worker must act on behalf of a client who has been adjudged legally incompetent, the social worker should safeguard the interests and rights of that client.
2. When another individual has been legally authorized to act in behalf of a client, the social worker should also deal with that person always with the client's best interests in mind.
3. The social worker should not engage in any action that violates or diminishes the civil or legal rights of clients. (1993, G, par. 1-3)

The first two obligations deal specifically with the rights of clients "legally adjudged" incompetent. The third deals with the civil and legal rights of all other clients.

Difficulties with the Code

Some practice situations, however, present us with dilemmas in implementing the principle that are not easily resolved. Some writers (Rothman, 1989; Keith-Lucas, 1975) have suggested that the traditional definitions of this principle, and even the Code itself, do not adequately address the reality of the practice situation. Keith-Lucas states that

> Self-determination should be in part conceived as a fact rather than a right, [and, in implementing self-determination] professionals are not respecting a right but acknowledging a reality within which meaningful helping activity must take place. (1975:2)

That is, self-determination is pragmatic. If the intervention of the social worker is to be successful it may well require the clients' help. This can hardly be obtained unless we recognize their active role. Rothman makes a closely related observation:

> The prime responsibility, therefore for making professional decisions about means of helping the client falls to the practitioner. . . . Nevertheless the helping process entails a joint relationship in which the client plays a significant but variable part. This suggests the principle of optimal client contributions to intervention planning. To the degree possible, the client should contribute actively to defining the difficulty to be addressed as well as the course of amelioration. *But the center of gravity, from the standpoint of structuring practice, lies with the professional rather than with the client.* (1989:608-609, emphasis added)

This balancing of our professional responsibility with our obligation to involve the clients to the maximum of their capacities in the helping process is the challenge of implementing this principle in practice. This chapter examines some aspects of that challenge.

PROFESSIONAL RESPONSIBILITY

Biestek spells out four main responsibilities of the worker in the implementation of the principle of self-determination with clients (1957:105-106). He was addressing practice with single clients but these obligations apply equally to work with multiclient systems.

First: To help the client see his or her problem or need clearly and with perspective. As noted earlier, we start always by accepting that the clients' definition of the problem is how it feels to this person, family, or group of people. This is the foundation of the helping relationship, and facilitates their looking at things from a different point of view, which we may offer for their consideration.

Second: To acquaint the client with the pertinent resources in the community. We need to inform clients about what may be available in the community to help them make their choice. For example, a woman who is trying to decide whether or not to leave an emotionally abusive husband and take the children to her parents' home in another state or province, needs to know that the Women's Centre in her city holds a free legal information clinic twice a month. There, an experienced family lawyer can give her clear, reliable information about her legal rights and the risks such a course of action could entail.

An organization of welfare recipients is determined to picket City Hall about what they see as discriminatory treatment by the municipal housing authority. They are made to wait for long periods in a public hallway where employees are constantly passing to and fro, engaging in loud conversations with much laughter. They may need to consider whether a small deputation to the housing authority might be more effective as a first step. They need, then, to know the specific person to whom that visit should be addressed.

In providing this kind of information, the worker must not oversell one course of action over another. We need to inform the clients, without pressure, what options are available. We need to clarify with the welfare recipients that as long as their demonstration is peaceful and not disruptive in any way, they do not run any legal risks. We also need, as stated in other chapters, to refrain from being "too helpful," taking over from the clients activities they are capable of doing for themselves. Such restraint on our part is empowering for clients, and helps them recognize that they have the freedom and the capacity to take action on their own behalf.

In some instances we may provide practical assistance–for example, our knowledge about the format of writing a grant proposal or other kind of formal request that may be part of a group's course of action in social action issues. This needs to be done in such a way that clients learn the technique, not that we "do it for" them. We must remember that imparting new skills for future problem solving is an integral part of effective help.

Third: To introduce stimuli that will activate the client's own dormant resources. Clients' resources may be "dormant" because of fear about the outcome of a course of action, and such fears may even prevent their realistically examining the plan. Clients may also be immobilized by fears that go a long way back in their personal experience and do not belong in the here and now. Some relevant stimuli may include the encouragement to examine the origin of the fear; support in regaining self-confidence about decision making, and help in looking objectively at the pros and cons of one action plan over another.

Fourth: To create a relationship environment in which the client can grow and work out his or her own problems. This is the essence of the concept of the social worker as partner and facilitator in the helping process. Biestek states that this facilitates the process whereby the client,

> using his own inner resources and the resources of the community, grows in the potential to work out his own problems, to move along at his own speed and in his own way. (1957:106)

SELF-DETERMINATION IN PRACTICE

Calvin, aged thirty-four, and Jeannette, aged thirty-three, came to the family service agency for marriage counseling. They said that until a few months ago their relationship has been relatively free of any serious conflict. However, in the last six months they have been quarreling seriously far more often, and frequently about what seem to them, in retrospect, rather trivial matters. Both really want to change this and to rebuild their relationship on a firm footing. They have two children, ages six and four. Jeannette works part-time outside the home in an insurance company. They bought a home at the time of their marriage eight years earlier.

In response to the worker's question, they reveal that six months ago, Jeannette's father began pressuring Calvin to come into his real estate business, as he wants to prepare for early retirement.

Calvin is an auto mechanic who works in the garage of a large car dealership where he has built up a solid reputation in ten years of steady employment. He enjoys his work, feels secure, and has a good benefit package. He has no interest in real estate, believes he would not be good in a sales job, and repeatedly says he is happy doing what he does now. He feels that Jeannette is pressuring him to make a change that is purely for her father's benefit, and is not taking his feelings into account.

Jeannette says that her father, aged fifty-nine, had a heart attack a year ago and made a good recovery, but wants to ease up on the pressures of his business and retire early. Her younger brother left the business four years ago to start his own computer company in another city, "for which my father has never forgiven him." She feels she and Calvin "owe" her father this deal because he lent them the down payment on their house, interest-free, as a wedding present, although they have paid it back in full. She says Calvin is being selfish to put his own job preference "ahead of everything."

In answer to the worker's question, she explains that "everything" to her means their relationship with her family and her parents' relationship with the grandchildren.

Calvin is obviously in distress while Jeannette is saying this. He says that he is trying to consider the change, for Jeannette's sake, but that he believes it is this that is causing the difficulties that lead to their quarreling. He believes it is important to him to enjoy what he does and he thinks real estate is not nearly as secure a living as his present employment.

Further exploration reveals that Jeannette's father was bitterly disappointed when, instead of going on to university to obtain a nursing degree, which he had been pushing her to do, she decided to follow her own interests—she went to a community college and obtained a diploma in accountancy. Apparently, her father barely spoke to her for several weeks after her decision and told her repeatedly that she had "let him down." She still remembers how dreadful it felt, at age eighteen, that he did not love her anymore. Her mother eventually took her side in this and the breach was healed. She led her class every year of the program, which helped.

Jeannette feels that her father was "disappointed" when she married Calvin, having hoped for a "lawyer or a doctor in the family." However, with a warm smile of pride she said that Calvin's obvious commitment to hard work, saving money, and what her father called "down-home values" won him over. She patted Calvin's knee and said, "Mom took to him right away." Jeannette says she wants Calvin to be happy, but cannot see why he couldn't make this change, for "everybody's sake." She added that she "couldn't bear it" if her Dad became ill again because of overwork.

At this point, Calvin reached over and took Jeannette's hand. Very near to tears he said, "Honey, I'm sorry you think I'm selfish, but I honestly don't think I'd be any good at sales and I believe it would make me unhappy, and I'm afraid I would blame you for it."

Discussion

It seems clear that most–perhaps all–of the tension between this couple is caused by the pressure from Jeannette's father for Calvin to change jobs.

Jeannette's seeming insistence on Calvin's making the change despite his wishes, and in spite of eight years of a relatively secure and happy marriage, may derive from the old pain of the consequences of her teenage defiance of her father. The worker will need to help her explore this.

It also raises one of the dilemmas that self-determination sometimes presents in practice, i.e., the right of one person in the client system over that of another.

The worker may have a definite preference in this case, on many rational grounds, for Calvin's refusing his father-in-law's demand. He will require vigilant self-awareness to ensure that he gives equal recognition to the reality of Jeannette's feelings and their influence on her perception of the situation.

The worker will need to facilitate the couple's exploration of the possible consequences of each course of action, and not to move in with what he may clearly see on the negative side. This is what Biestek calls a

> delicately balanced activity and passivity. The passivity consists of restraint in doing things *for and to the client,* thus helping the client to express himself as fully and freely as he wishes. (1957:105, emphasis added)

With the worker's sensitive help, this couple came to see that there were risks for their relationship and their children's security if Calvin made the change. It could seriously impair their overall well-being–personal, emotional, and possibly financial. Second, they recognized that they could not take responsibility for Jeannette's father's health by risking their own family's happiness and security. Jeannette identified her insistence on the plan as stemming from her eighteen-year-old despair at losing her father's love, but took some reassurance from her mother's support in the past, which had eventually won her father over.

Systems theory has taught us that any decision for change will inevitably have effects on others in the immediate social system (Levy, 1972:492). We need to help our clients examine and come to terms with those effects, as they struggle toward self-determination.

SELF-DETERMINATION WITH CHILDREN

We need to recognize that child-clients have the same right as adults to this principle. In many instances, children are involuntary candidates for our services, and their right to self-determination must be respected, as far as possible, within the framework of circumstances that bring them to us.

In child welfare agencies, for example, where a child's admission to care is voluntary on the part of the parent, it is important that the child's needs and wishes are not made subservient to the parent's or the agency's convenience, simply because this client is a child. School-age children who must make a move have their own business to attend to: a desk to be cleared out, goodbyes to be said to school friends, perhaps to a favorite teacher. As far as possible the child needs to be given some say in which day and at what time the move is made.

The same applies when a move must be made from one foster home to another. Sometimes even such minimal freedom as choosing whether they will move in the morning or afternoon can give the child some sense that he or she has some control over what is happening to them.

I believe we can show our respect for a very small child's right by asking, "Would you like to walk, or shall I carry you?" The car seat is an essential safety measure but a disadvantage is that a small child is removed from human touch at a time of stress. Wherever possible I believe that very young children should always be moved with two persons present, one to drive and the other to be with the child. This will include respecting his or her need for or rejection of comforting touch (hand-holding, for example) or verbal communication.[1]

SELF-DETERMINATION WITH GROUPS

The formation of a voluntary group requires a contract, often written, that defines the group's purpose and some rules of behavior–confidentiality within the group meetings, for example–to which everyone subscribes. The group worker acts as facilitator, but also models behavior for the group members, setting the example of respecting every member's contribution as being equally valuable to the group's purposes. Each member is heard, and we have a responsibility to ensure that they have been heard correctly.

Difficulties of various kinds can arise when one or more members want to exert a right of choice over the others. One or two members may attempt to take over, and develop a powerful clique that can divert the group's purpose and ultimately destroy the group. This has to be recognized very early, and brought out into the open; everyone's feelings about it need to be sought and respectfully recognized.

Another difficulty can arise when the need of one member gets in the way of the group's working to achieve its overall objective.

> In a voluntary group of nine girls, twelve to fourteen years of age, in agency foster and group home care, the worker suggested that the group might consider its purpose as sharing feelings about being "in care." Some members suggested an

important issue for them was difficulty with family relationships, about visits with parents and/or not wanting visits; others wanted relationships with boys included. The group consensus was that relationships with family and sharing feelings
about being in care were their most immediate concerns; relationships with boys were not really a priority.

The worker explained that they all needed to accept the
responsibility to keep everything that was said in the group
meetings completely confidential; without this, no one would
feel safe to share her real feelings. There was some discussion
about this, and whether they could trust each other. Heather
asked if that applied to the worker as well. Would she tell their
own primary worker or their foster or group home parents
what they had said here? The worker explained that she was
professionally bound not to divulge anything to any other person, without the girl's consent. Heather said she guessed they
had to take that on faith. The worker said she would be fired if
she betrayed their confidence, but, yes, until they got to know
each other better, she had to ask them to take it on faith.

Early in the second meeting, Laurel, age twelve, said she
wanted to talk about a problem she was having with a new
boyfriend. He was coming on very strong about having sex,
and was very angry when she refused. She didn't know how to
handle it. She liked the boy, and was afraid of losing him if she
said no, but she is still a virgin and is not sure if she wants to
start having sex yet. Heather said Laurel could not take up the
group's time with that—it had been agreed that boyfriend issues
were not the first priority. Laurel looked very downcast. Margo
said she felt that the group should be prepared to put their own
concerns aside for part of the meeting to help Laurel because
"lots of us have been there and we know how it feels." There
was a murmur of agreement from several other members.

Karen asked the worker what she thought. The worker said
it was up to the group to decide. Ashley, a very quiet girl, said
she thought it was a pity if the group's meetings had to be like
"business meetings" with an agenda that could not be
changed. Heather asked what was the point of having set priorities if they didn't stick to them. Margo suggested that they

ask at the beginning of each meeting if anyone had something really urgent that was not about family or foster care, and that some time be allocated for these issues at each meeting. Karen suggested that they schedule one meeting a month for boy-friend issues only. The members talked over these suggestions for a while, occasionally asking the worker to intervene and decide. The worker refused, saying that she thought they were debating the point very responsibly and she had confidence they could work things out the best way for everyone. She intervened once, when one girl told another that her remark was "childish and stupid," reminding them that everyone's voice must be respectfully heard here.

Finally Karen said she believed they were wrong in not letting Laurel talk about her problem because it was obviously pressing; they could think about the question of if, when, and how to be flexible, and bring back ideas for a decision at the next meeting. Everyone agreed, and Laurel began to talk about her difficulty. The worker noted that nearly all the girls, even those who had initially opposed this move, took an active part in a very responsible, and for the most part, sensitive way of talking about Laurel's struggle. She commended the group on the way they had handled this difficulty.

Discussion

This issue of one member's right to assert his or her need over the group's right as a whole to stick to their own agenda is not always resolved as readily as in this example. The worker needs to balance his or her intervention between active participation and allowing the group to move in its own way (Behroozi, 1992:103), and, as in the example given, the group will often manage very well with its own decision making. Practice in making such choices assists the development within members of the tools of self-determination.

In some instances, the worker may need to define this last aspect of his or her professional responsibility explicitly.

A family service agency was sponsoring a voluntary group of seven young single men, all survivors of childhood sexual abuse. The purpose of the group had been agreed upon as sharing and coming to terms with their feelings about the abuse. All members agreed that these feelings often got in the way of their relationships with parents, girlfriends, and in the workplace.

Quite early in the group's progress, Colin began to take an informal leadership role, questioning members about their contributions in an aggressive way and offering unsought advice. He did not share his own personal experiences or feelings. The other members seemed intimidated by Colin. More than once the worker invited a member to tell Colin how his comment made him feel, but no one really responded. Colin did not "take the hint" from the worker's interventions.

After the third meeting, Mark and Robert stayed to talk to the worker about their feelings about Colin, and said that unless he changed they wanted him out of the group. The worker acknowledged the difficulty and explained that he thought this was a matter for the group to deal with; that it was important for them all and for Colin that they help him see that his behavior was destructive to the fulfillment of the group's objectives. Mark and Robin said they had canvassed the members since the last meeting and all had agreed that the worker should talk privately to Colin about it.

The worker refused to do this, and discussed with them how they might begin to deal with this at the next meeting.

Discussion

This example shows the worker's dilemma in such a situation. Clearly Colin's behavior is disruptive. His right of self-determination cannot be given precedence over the rights of the group. In many ways it would be easier for everyone, perhaps especially Colin, if the worker agreed to the plan offered by the troubled members. The worker's choice to give it back to the group offers them a learning experience about confronting a situation in which their self-esteem—one of the most critical issues for such men—is threatened.

This case illustrates the importance of our holding firmly to our professional responsibility, where the easy way out appears to contribute to everyone's comfort. "Do you want to be nice, or do you want to be helpful?" one beginning worker was asked by his supervisor (Lamb, 1995:4). Weick and Pope remind us that professional helping is built on the assumption that

> the central task of every human is to become more fully and more uniquely him or herself; its goal is growth, not happiness. (1988:16)

We must ensure that as far possible all our interventions contribute to that growth.

SELF-DETERMINATION IN COMMUNITY PRACTICE

Implementing self-determination can present some special difficulties in this field of practice. Fundamentally the issues are of course the same: the question of legality of any course of action, consideration of the rights of others, acceptance of the rights of all members of the group to be heard and to participate, and contributing to the achievement of the community group's purpose.

The organization of welfare recipients mentioned earlier, whose first plan of action was to picket City Hall as a way of making their wants known, may or may not agree to the worker's suggestion that a small deputation to the housing authority might be a more effective first step. As long as their demonstration is orderly and does not disrupt street or sidewalk traffic, there could be no legal consequences for them if they choose to picket.

Despite the worker's conviction that this will be less effective in the long run, it is the group's right to find out for themselves whether or not this is true. It is also quite possible that the worker is wrong, and that the publicity of a street protest will act as a shock treatment to get things moving.[2]

What matters is that people feel free to choose the plan that makes most sense to them; that they have not been told by "experts" what is good for them, and that they can find out for themselves what works and what does not.

Social Assistance department staff have contacted the Outreach Division of a psychiatric hospital in the east end of a large city about their concern for a number of discharged patients residing in the surrounding low-income area. These men and women are receiving social assistance and disability pensions, and living in low-cost rooming and boarding houses.

The Social Assistance workers state that they believe there is a need for a drop-in center for these clients, in a readily accessible, neutral location. Ideally a psychiatric social worker from the hospital would be on duty, but it is possible that the local branch of the Mental Health Association could offer volunteers whom the hospital staff could train. A social worker from the hospital could come in part-time. The objective could be primarily recreational with personal consultation available, and some group work could be done (if the clients were willing) around recovery and rehabilitation issues.

The hospital administration agreed that this was a possibility and they would explore funding. Social Services staff would also explore this with the city, and felt that a start-up grant could be forthcoming.

It was agreed that the social workers would suggest a meeting with any clients who were interested. A local church offered its hall for this purpose. Several clients responded that they would not come to a meeting at the church; two were Muslims and four others said they "wanted nothing to do with religion." Eventually the meeting was held in a small meeting room at the Public Health Unit offices; the clients agreed that after hours there would be no other people around who might "wonder–and start gossiping."

When the drop-in center was put to the group, there was at first no response. Encouraged to offer their ideas, two of the men said they had been talking with some of the group about changing things for themselves, and put forward the idea that they use this money to work up part of a long-time vacant lot at the end of a nearby street to grow flowers and vegetables.[3] These men said that the gardening they did while in hospital had really made them feel good, and several others, both men and women, agreed.

As the discussion proceeded it became clear that the gardening idea caught the imagination of a majority of this group. They considered it was more important for them than a drop-in center; it was late February and they would need to get something going if the garden was to become a reality this year. As far as they were concerned, the drop-in center could wait until the winter when there was nothing to do.

They planned to work the garden as a cooperative, and to sell flowers and fresh vegetables either on the street or to local convenience stores. One of the women had already talked to her landlady, who had offered the loan of gardening tools. They told the workers they would need their help with the necessary formalities—a grant proposal to the city to get started, street-vending permits, and so on. Four of them have already started a clean-up on the vacant lot as a measure of good faith.

Discussion

It is clear that the drop-in center cannot be imposed on this group of people. Their preference for the gardening project as a means of improving their life circumstances is clear. Everyone's interests—including both agencies'—are better served by allowing them to determine what is, in their view, more important for their well-being. While the workers will need to be realistic about obstacles that may arise, they will need to demonstrate their commitment to these clients' right of self-determination in their support of and practical help with the plan.[4]

LIMITATIONS

While we must in all cases proceed from the base of our commitment to self-determination, there are realistic limitations on this right. As noted earlier, Biestek, among others, cites, for example, the client's capacity for positive and constructive decision making; the criminal, civil, and moral law; the rights of others; and the rights of the agency.

Limitations of Client Capacity

Biestek notes that the age and mental competence of the client may impose realistic limitations on the implementation of this right

(1957:110-112). This may apply in work with children and with the mentally challenged, but it is also a significant factor in work with the physically ill and elders, whether in the community or in hospitals. Sometimes we must make a decision for the client in such instances, or we may need to advise and help others who have assumed or been legally given that decision-making responsibility.

Several writers on this subject (Bennett, 1988; Kapp, 1988; Nicholson and Matross, 1989; and Soskis and Kerson, 1992) remind us that the assumption from the start must be that clients have the necessary capacity or "competence" to make sound decisions for their own well-being. Where it is determined that clients do not have such capacity, there is legal provision in most jurisdictions for another person or persons to take charge and make the decision on the clients' behalf. In making such decisions the ruling factor must be the clients' "best interests" in terms that take into account their total mental, physical, psychological, and social condition.

When individuals refuse to accept services, we must not take such refusal at face value. We need to ensure that they have adequate information and to explain fully and clearly, in terms the persons can understand, just what is involved in their accepting or refusing the service (Kapp, 1988:3). Having made such explanations as clearly as we can, we must still bear in mind what Nicholson and Matross say:

> The ethical principle of autonomy and the legal tenet of informed consent prohibit forcing competent patients to undergo any treatment against their will, even for their own good. (1989:234)

Kapp distinguishes between the imposition of services that others consider desirable for the person, and those that are considered necessary (1988:1-5). He points out that in some cases community health and well-being must take precedence and services must be imposed on an individual who is refusing them. He cites the example of a woman whose twenty-six cats in a small apartment posed a threat to her neighbors' health (1988:3-4).

In instances where only the individual's well-being is at stake, the primary issue in overruling their refusal of service is that of determining when a client's competence is not adequate for making a decision that has life-changing effects. Kapp points out that

> there is no unanimity or precision as to defining [competence] or applying tests. Thus the burden of proof rests with those who seek to challenge or [over-rule a person's capacity] in such situations. (1988:5)

There is general agreement that the concept of competence is relative, not absolute, suggesting that "an individual is competent if she is able to decide not well, but well enough" (Kapp, 1988:5). Bennett states that social workers need to

> accept the idea of limited or partial decision-making capacity in clients. Since competence is a relative quality, an individual may be able to make a specific decision, but be limited in other areas. (1988:16)

In estimating client competence, we can get some guidance from the President's Commission criteria, notably:

- possession of a set of values and goals,
- the ability to communicate and understand information, and
- the ability to reason and deliberate about one's choices. (cited in Nicholson and Matross, 1989:234)

Even the guidance of these criteria, however, leave difficult decisions about the rationality of a given choice. We need to take account of the total situation of the person making that decision. Kapp cites as an example that

> an elderly individual choosing short-term comfort over long-term survival may not be acting irrationally—a younger, otherwise vibrant person making the same decision would seem irrational in the helping profession's value scheme. (1988:6)

As noted earlier, some jurisdictions recognize the validity of living wills, advance directives, or health care proxy statements, in which individuals, at a time when their capacity is not impaired, state how they wish to be treated in the event of failing capacity. These are dealt with in detail in Soskis and Kerson's (1992) valuable discussion of the U.S. Federal 1991 Patient Self-Determination Act. These writers also emphasize that social workers have special responsibilities in the Act's implementation.

The legislation varies from one jurisdiction to another in defining and restricting the circumstances and the manner in which someone may be empowered to make a decision for another individual. In his detailed discussion of the need for intervention by others in taking over decision-making power, Kapp (1988) cites Cohen (1986), who states that such interventions should be governed by the "principle of the least restrictive or least invasive alternative." Further elaboration on these complex matters is not appropriate here.

Discussion of other kinds of limitations can be usefully divided into their application of agency rights in work with voluntary and involuntary clients.

AGENCY RIGHTS

Voluntary Clients

In counseling voluntary clients, we may sometimes be faced with a conflict between the clients' wishes about how the service is to be offered, and the agency's professional responsibility.

For example, family service agencies are committed to whole-family therapy, because it has been amply demonstrated to be both theoretically sound and pragmatically effective. As stated in an earlier chapter, a couple who brings a rebellious teenager to the agency as "the problem to be fixed" will be informed about the agency's policy and the reasons for it. This couple does not have the right to determine how the service will be offered in their case. They only have the right to choose whether or not they will accept the service. It would be unethical for the agency to be flexible in this, in that everything we know about family therapy tells us that separating the family members for intervention is unhelpful.

A similar instance may occur in a child welfare agency with a runaway child. The nature of the child's complaints, his or her stated reasons for running away, and of course his or her age all affect the child's right. If the child is legally a "child" within the jurisdiction in which service is being offered, and if there does not appear to be any physical or sexual abuse, the parents must be involved at the first opportunity. The child does not, in such instances, have the right to refuse this.

The worker's skill in handling such contact is the critical factor here. Sensitivity to the feelings of both child and parents, adherence to principles of acceptance, and a nonjudgmental attitude and skill in building a professional relationship on the basis of these persons' current reality will all be crucial to reuniting the family more securely.

As noted earlier, most adoption agencies require couples applying to adopt children to attend one or more group meetings of applicants as part of the adoption procedure. Again, this procedure has been shown to help couples examine the real life meaning of adoption and to share their hopes and fears with others considering the same decision. Since such groups have demonstrated their effectiveness the agency has the right to require these clients to attend.

Vocational rehabilitation services, under public or private auspices, are offered to a voluntary clientele. However, it is usually a condition of the service that clients consent to a contact with their physician for a complete medical history and assessment. Without this, the service will not–indeed cannot–be provided. In all the above instances the consequences of the decision not to accept service need to be clearly discussed with the client.

Involuntary Candidates

Behroozi (1992) and Goldstein (1986) discuss in detail the ethical and practice issues of work with persons who have not chosen to come for service, but have done so under some external pressure. This may be a probation order, where an offender's probation terms include attendance at a therapy group designed for their specific problem. They may come to us under a child welfare court order–for example, abusive or negligent parents, or runaway adolescents. Behroozi calls these persons "involuntary applicants"[5] and reminds us that our first job is to help them move to client status, i.e., voluntary membership in the social work group.

The worker here needs to accept the person's reluctance as understandable; to create an atmosphere of trust that each person in the group will be heard, understood, and not judged, and to point out the advantages to their making changes in their behavior. As noted earlier, I believe we do not need to look for one hundred percent acceptance of the value of group attendance in every member of this group of clients. I believe that "I guess I've got to give it a try" is an adequate beginning.

Reluctance can have many causes (Behroozi 1992:227). A majority of these persons are the economically and/or ethnically disadvantaged or marginalized members of our communities. Clients' reluctance to enter into a group work contract in these circumstances may be their way of making a "last stand" for control over their own lives. It may also reflect feelings of failure and incompetence, and/or rage against a society that has never listened to their needs or supported their aspirations. Lastly, we need to take into account that many of these people have had bad experiences with authority in the past, and may feel that we represent "a system that has been their adversary" (Riordan, Matheny, and Harris, cited in Behroozi, 1992:226).

The circumstances of these persons coming for service place unalterable limits on their right of self-determination. Behroozi points out that this creates an ethical problem for workers, a "Double Bind" in which we feel caught between the rights of the clients and the mandate of the agency (1992:224-225). The workers' problem is

> how to reconcile their professional obligations to [this group of persons] with the requirements of their employing institutions. (1992:225)

A way of resolving this dilemma is cited by Garvin who states that social group work services in social control settings

> complement the institution's social control function by helping group members to meet their own needs in socially acceptable ways. (1987:254-255)

However, Garvin further states that the interests of the clients must not be totally subservient to the mission of the agency (1987:255).

Workers need to look for opportunities for participants in these groups to exercise as much of their right of self-determination as is compatible with the terms of whatever legal requirement has placed them there. Sound group work practice, within the legal framework, can ensure that the principle is implemented appropriately.

Legal Limitations

Voluntary or involuntary clients may come to us with a plan of action that conflicts with a civil or criminal law. It is vital that we acquaint them fully with the risk of legal consequences they run into when choosing to engage in such a plan. Biestek cites the example of a divorced, noncustodial parent who was planning to abduct his child and take him into another state (1957:114-115). In a case such as this we have a responsibility to help the client recognize not only the legal consequences, but also to consider the emotional effects such an action would have on his child. In some instances, as noted earlier, we may be legally obliged to break confidentiality.

The Rights of Others

We may see voluntary or involuntary clients who want to pursue a course of action that infringes the rights of others. We have an obligation to express concern about any such plan. We need to help the client see what are the rights of others in the particular situation and what harm—emotional or other—can result from the client's following his or her own will.

Limitations of Conscience of Worker or Client

Biestek cites one more category of limitation on client self-determination, i.e., matters of conscience (1957:116-118). This can arise with voluntary or involuntary clients where there is a difference of religious conviction between worker and client.

> A young woman coming to a nondenominational family service agency complaining of a "family problem" is assigned to a Catholic worker. Exploration reveals that the client is eigh-

teen years old, and has recently split up with a boyfriend with whom she has lived for almost a year. When she told him she was pregnant, he left and moved out of the state. Abortion is legal in the jurisdiction where she and the agency are located. The client belongs to a Protestant denomination that accepts abortion. She needs advice about where she can obtain the procedure. In such a situation the worker must explain her own position on abortion to the client and that she cannot advise a course of action that is against her religious beliefs. Taking care to interpret the referral as sensitively as possible, the worker must arrange a transfer to another staff member for whom this is not a problem of conscience.[6]

A similar difficulty may arise when the client is also Catholic but wishes to obtain an abortion despite the teachings of her faith. A Protestant worker who accepts abortion will need to discuss with the client that when the perceived crisis of unwanted pregnancy is resolved, the client may suffer considerable guilt and stress. It will be appropriate to discuss alternatives fully, so that this client can make a considered decision.[7]

Biestek says that

> To help client[s] remain true to [themselves] in times of stress, when [they are] tempted to violate [their] own principles is a great service to [them]. (1957:117)

In today's multicultural, multifaith communities, we shall often find ourselves facing dilemmas of this kind.

In conclusion, the practical implementation of this principle clearly requires of us the most careful attention to the recognition of the boundaries, in each case, between the clients' right to self-determination and our professional responsibility for helping them to achieve healthy outcomes.

SUMMARY OF MAIN POINTS

1. The right of client self-determination is both a value and a method principle and an essential component of sound professional helping.

2. Limitations on this right, however, are imposed by legal requirements, the agency's mandate and/or policies, the rights of others, and the client's age and mental capacity.
3. There is a strong argument for considering self-determination as a fact with which we must come to terms, rather than a right that we must be concerned to "grant."
4. We must make clear to clients those limitations that apply in their particular situation.
5. We have a responsibility to help clients examine their difficulty objectively.
6. Genuine choice for clients requires that they are fully informed of what community resources may be available for them.
7. We must create a climate of trust in which clients feel safe to explore and develop their own potential for problem solving.
8. We must always facilitate the clients' full examination of the consequences for them and for others of any course of action they want to take.
9. We must always bear in mind that child-clients are entitled to this right to the maximum that their age, capacity, and legal status allow.
10. We need to respect the feelings of those who are required by some legal decree to accept services not of their own choosing. Within the limits of the legal requirements, we must provide opportunities for them to exercise their right of self-determination wherever and whenever possible.
11. The clients' conscience, or our own, may be a factor to be taken into account in their decision making and our support of their choice.

NOTES

1. Students may want to discuss the implication of current concerns about "inappropriate touching" on this traditional adult-to-child comforting responsibility.

2. This might well be true, especially in a small city where local media publicity could carry considerable weight.

3. This case was introduced in the chapter on Individualization.

4. This case may appear unrealistic in light of today's funding cutback policies. It is included because I believe it illustrates the principle effectively. Class-

room discussion of the effect of policy restrictions on the worker's role in this situation could be fruitful.

5. I prefer to call them "candidates" (see Chapter 1), since their eligibility for service has been determined by external forces.

6. Clients generally experience such a referral as rejection.

7. It is recognized that members of many other faiths will share this difficulty.

REFERENCES

Behroozi, Cyrus S. (1992). "A Model for Social Work Practice with Involuntary Applicants in Groups." *Social Work with Groups*, 15(2-3):223-238.

Bennett, Claire. (1988). "A Social Worker Comments: Some Implications for Social Work Practice in Health Settings." *Social Work in Health Care,* 3(4):15-18.

Biestek, Felix P. (1957). *The Casework Relationship.* Chicago, IL: Loyola University Press.

Cohen, Elias S. (1986). "Nursing Homes and the Least Restrictive Environment Doctrine." In Marshall B. Kapp, Harvey E. Pies, and A. Edward Doudera, eds. *Legal and Ethical Aspects of Health Care for the Elderly.* Ann Arbor, MI: Health Administration Press.

Dolgoff, Ralph and Louise Skolnik. (1992). "Ethical Decision-Making, the NASW Code of Ethics and Group Work Practice." *Social Work with Groups*, 15(4):99-112.

Garvin, Charles. (1987). *Contemporary Group Work, Second Edition.* Englewood Cliffs, NJ: Prentice-Hall.

Goldstein, Howard. (1986). "A Cognitive-Humanistic Approach to the Hard-to-Reach Client." *Social Casework*, 67(1):27-36.

Kapp, Marshall B. (1988). "Forcing Services on At-Risk Older Adults: When Doing Good Is Not So Good." *Social Work in Health Care*, 13(4):1-13.

Keith-Lucas, Alan. (1975). "A Critique of the Principle of Client Self-Determination." In *Self-Determination in Social Work.* F.E. McDermott, ed. London: Routledge and Keegan Paul. Cited in J. Rothman, 1989.

Lamb, Bill. (1995). Tribute to the late Dr. Stan Skarsten. *IFL Reflections.* Toronto, Canada: The Institute of Family Living (Spring).

Levy, Charles S. (1972). "Values and Planned Change." *Social Casework*, 53(10):488-493.

National Association of Social Workers. (1993). *Code of Ethics of the National Association of Social Workers.* Washington, DC: NASW.

Nicholson, Barbara and Gerald Matross. (1989). "Facing Reduced Decision-Making in Health Care: Methods for Maintaining Client Self-Determination." *Social Work*, 34(3):234-238.

President's 1983 Commission for the Study of Ethical Problems in Medicine and Biomedical and Behavioral Research. *Deciding to Forego Life-Sustaining Treatment: A Report of the Ethical, Medical, and Moral Issues in Treatment*

Decisions. Washington, DC: Government Printing Office. Cited in Nicholson and Matross, 1989.

Riordan, Richard J., Kenneth Matheny, and Charles M. Harris. (1989). "Helping Counsellors Minimize Client Reluctance." *Counsellor Education and Supervision*, 18:7-13.

Rothman, J. (1989). "Client Self-Determination: Untangling the Knot." *Social Service Review*, 63(4):598-612.

Soskis, Carole W. and Toba Schwaber Kerson. (1992). "The Patient Self-Determination Act." *Social Work in Health Care*, 16(4):1-18.

Weick, Ann and Loren Pope. (1988). "Knowing What's Best: A New Look at Self-Determination." *Social Casework*, 69(1):10-16.

OTHER USEFUL READING

Freedberg, Sharon. (1989). "Self-Determination: Historical Perspectives and Effects on Current Practice." *Social Work*, 34(1):33-38.

Chapter 12

Involvement of the Client in the Helping Process: Sharing the Work of Change

This principle is implicit in much of what is contained in several other chapters in this text. However, it merits some specifically focused discussion because effective help requires that we consciously build it into our practice method.

In an earlier chapter, social work was defined as a goal-oriented undertaking between persons who desire change or are under some external pressure to bring about change in human situations, and other persons whose position and training designate them as agents of change. Clearly this is a "mutual endeavor, in which both parties share responsibility for making change happen" (Corey and Corey, 1993:63). Thus the helping process lays certain role obligations upon both participants.

THE WORKER'S ROLE

It is useful here to repeat the earlier stated three essential ingredients of the helping process; they define, in broad terms, the role obligations of the worker. These are

- the resolution or significant amelioration of the presenting problem(s), in such a way that
- the client's self-esteem is healed and/or enhanced and his/her psychosocial growth promoted, and that
- new skills and tools of coping are learned that enhance his/her capacity to meet life demands more effectively in the future.

THE CLIENT'S ROLE

In an early chapter it was noted that applicants or candidates for service become clients when

- they recognize a need for change;
- they accept us as a source of help for change; and
- they become willing to involve themselves in the process of change.

This is in essence the person's or group's acceptance of the role of client. Discussing the role of "client" as distinct, for example, from that of "patient," Siporin says:

> A client generally retains much more active responsibility and autonomy in relation to the helping agent, and is expected to assume active, task-performing roles in the helping process. (1975:179)

As noted earlier, the nature of social work help requires that the client share personal facts, thoughts, and feelings that relate to their trouble. Clients are also expected to be responsible in keeping appointments, and in payment of fees, where this is applicable (Siporin, 1975:180-181.) Social workers are also required to be responsible about scheduling and keeping appointments.

The sharing of the task begins at the first contact, and continues throughout the process until the desired change is, at some satisfactory level, achieved. It is integral to the processes of study, assessment, and implementing the intervention plan. The role obligations of both partners in the progress of the helping process will be highlighted in the following discussion.

STUDY AND ASSESSMENT PHASE

The kind of sharing that needs to take place in study and assessment comprises the clients' view of the presenting problem together with how it appears to us from the professional view. As the work progresses, both these views may be amended as new information is shared, but the sooner both participants begin to discern patterns in the problem's manifestations, the more effectively they will be able to think about possible solutions to the problems.

Clients are the experts about how they experience their problem as individuals, families, or groups of persons. The worker's role is first to create the climate of trust in which clients can meet their role obligation to share with us–in their own way, as openly and honestly as possible–how the problem feels, what they think about it, and how they perceive it. As noted earlier, all of these are integral to the total reality of their situation, which also includes how they feel about not being able to resolve the problem without outside help, and how they feel about us and the particular auspices under which we are offering them a helping service. We may also need to take into account ethnic and cultural aspects of their feelings about needing and accepting our help. As noted in an earlier chapter, they may feel resentment and humiliation if they are involuntary candidates in an authority-based setting. This "allows the worker and client to gain a beginning sense of the interplay of forces within the client's life-space" (Germain and Gitterman, 1980:47).

This sharing will often require that they disclose painful material–perhaps thoughts, feelings, or actions of which they have been ashamed. If we listen and respond to their stories with acceptance and without negative judgment, we will convey our recognition that they know more about how it feels to experience their troubles than we do. This also communicates a basic respect that can be reassuring to their self-worth.

Our next role obligation is to bring to their stories our knowledge of human behavior and our empathic understanding of them as individuals, families, or groups in their own social milieu; we must share our knowledge and understanding with them in ways that will respect their individuality, as well as accept them as persons. As noted earlier, the judgments we need to make should only concern their behavior, thinking, and attitudes, and how these relate to the problem. We also need to verbalize how these may identify strengths or areas of difficulty for this person, family, or group. It is worth repeating here that these judgments are made strictly in the context of assessment, not of condemnation.

We cannot determine the validity of any part of our assessment without checking it out with the clients; we need to ascertain whether or not they understand and accept the premise and/or line of reasoning that may result from the assessment. We need to be sure that our view of the problem makes sense to them.

Despite our knowledge and insight, it is very important that we do not "push" or rush into offering early interpretation. Someone has written, "let the client do the work," and we need to remember that if clients, at their own pace, arrive at a different perception of their difficulties, they have perhaps made their first use of what can become a tool for looking at future difficulties in a new way.

The Use of Homework Assignments

This is an important way of involving clients actively in the course of the helping process. In study and assessment these can vary a great deal. They need to be geared to the particular client's or group member's level of functioning, cognitive abilities, and so on. For some clients the making of a family genogram is useful (Germain and Gitterman, 1980:114,239). This seeks to identify relationships between all family members, including those in close touch and any who are estranged. It may also identify, where appropriate, those members with alcohol problems, criminal records, and so on.

After they have been taught reflective listening in a session, couples in conflict may be asked to set a time once a week—perhaps Sunday evening—in which they practice taking turns talking about their feelings about certain events or exchanges during the week, without any interruptions or immediate responses from the other. Each in turn then reflects back what they have heard, without any personal comment or evaluation, to ensure that they have heard correctly what was being expressed. This can illuminate a problem for the couple in that they can begin to recognize how little attention they customarily pay to trying to hear what the other is really saying. Reporting one of these exercises, one client told the worker "I realized that while Kelly's talking about her feelings, I'm always just waiting to get in my two cents' worth."

For some clients in the study and assessment phase and/or later in the process, it can be useful to assign written homework. After painful material has been examined, or after there has been an unresolved difference of viewpoint between worker and client, thought-ful journal writing about how clients felt following the interview can be very helpful. As indicated in an earlier case example illustrating release of feelings, others can be encouraged to write letters to an abusive or neglectful parent; these are letters that will never be mailed, but only read and reviewed with the worker. Some survivors of sexual abuse, or some adult children of alcoholics may be offered appropriate self-help books to read.

In considering the assignment of such tasks, we need to examine very carefully the individual client's or family's capacities and inter-ests. We may believe that a certain self-help book could help Sharon understand that she is not alone in feeling to blame for her brother's sexual abuse. If Sharon is not in the habit of gaining anything from reading, our suggestion will be of no help. On the contrary, it will only lead her to believe that we just "don't understand how it feels."

When clients have been unable to complete a written assignment I have found it very useful to discuss the reasons why it was diffi-cult, or impossible. If a relationship of trust has been built, and if they see that their failure to complete the assignment is accepted as a difficulty for them, and not for me, sensitive discussion can be very helpful. It can illuminate an aspect of the difficulty that had not previously come to light. Germain and Gitterman state that "[cli-ents] need the worker's support, but not the burden of pleasing her" (1980:239).

Timing is also very important. We must take into consideration the client's readiness for any task we might suggest. While a part of that readiness lies within our responsibility for focusing the inter-views and maintaining a goal orientation, the client's individual pace of working must be a concern—again we need to watch that we do not "push" for our pace rather than move at theirs.

This kind of pressure usually arises only from our genuine desire to help, but we need to guard against it, nonetheless. For many years I have had the following admonition in full view on my desk: "It is so much easier to tell a person what to do with his problem than to stand with him in his pain" (David Augsburger, date and source unknown).

While working with families, relationship problems can sometimes be usefully illustrated through giving experiential tasks, such as "sculpting." This is a way of helping family members experience physically the kind of relationships that trouble them.

> The Zavitz family were in counseling because of the troubled relationships between the parents and their three young teenage children. Carl, aged fifteen, had at first been identified by the family as the most troubled one, but through counseling they had begun to realize that the difficulties were much more general.
>
> They agreed to a sculpting exercise, and the worker suggested that Carl start directing the positioning of the family members. Father was directed by Carl to sit on a chair alone, facing the rest of the family, but at some distance from them. The other children agreed solidly with this. Asked by the worker how he felt about this position, Father said, half-humorously, that it felt "safe." Mother was directed to take a position standing facing him, and she voluntarily stretched her arms out toward Father. The three children stood close, all touching her. They looked at Father, but made no gestures toward him.
>
> When asked by the worker if this position expressed how she felt, Mother said, "No! The children should be on the floor, so I can feel the weight of them dragging on me." The children sat down on the floor, and hung on to her arms. Tearfully Mother said to Father, "Can't you SEE this is how it's always been, ever since the children began to grow up?"
>
> This helped to create a breakthrough in this highly motivated family's acknowledgement of who was troubled and why. Mr. Zavitz's father had deserted his family when he was four years old. He had been good with the children as babies and toddlers, but when they began to assert themselves he withdrew emotionally from them and his wife. Family therapy proceeded successfully thereafter through open and genuine communication.

A more concrete—and perhaps less threatening—way for some clients to realize the patterns of dysfunctional family relationships can be achieved using small blocks of wood of various sizes. Blocks of different sizes can be selected to represent each family member—

sometimes illustrating their importance or power in the family. They can then be placed by each family member in positions of relationship–close or at a distance–that illustrate their "fit" in the family's configuration, as seen by the member who is doing the model. This can illuminate the troubled relationships in the family and can form a constructive basis for discussion. It can also be used with single adult clients struggling to come to terms with disturbed family relationships, or those who are recovering from physical or emotional childhood abuse (Middleton-Moz, 1994).

Some clients may decide that their comfort and well-being in the workplace requires that they deal openly with a colleague who is causing them distress. Rehearsing with clients how they will deal with this–either through actual written excerpts, careful notetaking, or addressing the "empty chair"–can be constructively helpful. One client dictated to me what she really wanted to say. We then went over it and made changes that helped her stick to facts, making it more acceptable, and not leaving her open to accusations of trouble-making or bad temper. She took it home and rehearsed it by herself, made some changes, and went over it once again with me. She handled the interview at her place of work very capably and with good results.

Task-Assignment with Groups

In working for the achievement of a group's purpose, workers need to maintain a certain level of participation from all group members. Workers have a responsibility to make this expectation clear from the outset, and they need to model the kind of openness, attentiveness to feelings, and respectful response that can be important for the group members to learn. The group's purpose–whether it is learning, personal growth, or social action–will only be achieved if the worker creates the climate in which the members can interact constructively in this way.

In some groups (depending on the purpose) role-playing may be appropriate. It can bring a sense of reality, in a safe setting, wherein members can reenact troubled interactions. It can help both those who take part in the role-playing and those who observe and share in discussion afterwards.

Implementing the Action Plan

Regardless of the number of persons in the client group, the implementation of action plans needs to be thoughtfully worked out between worker and clients. In determining who does what, we need to take into account their conviction about the worthwhileness of the plan; this requires free and open discussion to determine, for example in a community action group, if there is a strong feeling that the plan is worth trying. Second, we need to assess how pessimistic are those people who do not believe it will work. It may be possible to work out a compromise that is more agreeable and supported by the group as whole. If not, a new plan needs to be developed. Our readiness to accept all points of view is an important factor in achieving goals.

We must also take into account the capacities of the clients, both in terms of their personal and practical abilities, their verbal skills, transportation issues, and any previous experience they may have had in contacting community leaders or officials who need to be approached. All need to be considered. We need to examine with our clients who is the best person or group to take on certain parts of the action plan. We must also help them assess the level of their confidence that they can carry out those parts of the task, and take the likelihood of success into account. A "small" success is not really so small; it can be a starting point for clients to build self-confidence in taking charge of their lives.

In action-oriented community groups, action plans need to be carefully reviewed with the group, and a suitable division of labor between worker and client group needs to be worked out. For example, a neighborhood action group that wants to conduct an education project about racism may have contacts within the community who are more accessible to certain group members than they are to the worker. The worker, on the other hand, may have more access to funding sources, and may be able to make more suggestions concerning the design and implementation of the program.

As noted earlier, it is important that the community's action plans are realistic and presented in a manner that increases their likelihood of being listened to and taken seriously by the persons or organizations to which they are addressed. This will be discussed in detail under the heading of Empowerment, but we need to remember that teaching these skills is a part of our responsibility.

Our professional commitment to effective helping lays upon us the responsibility to involve our clients actively in the helping process from beginning to termination. Finding ways to do this—whether working with individuals, couples, families, groups, or in communities—challenges both our creativity and our practical skills of relating to people from different backgrounds and in various social and political contexts.

SUMMARY OF MAIN POINTS

1. Professional helping is by definition a shared process; both client and worker are responsible for achieving a desired outcome.
2. These responsibilities can be identified as role obligations, and they apply regardless of the numerical size of the client system.
3. The first element of the worker's role is to create a climate of respect and trust in which clients can feel it is safe to meet the first obligation of their role—sharing their story—in an open way.
4. Clients know more about how they experience their struggles than we do. We share with them our knowledge of human behavior and our empathic understanding of their difficulty.
5. As we share this, we need to check out whether or not our view makes sense to the clients. This consistent sharing of input moves the process through study and assessment toward the development of an action plan to resolve the problem.
6. Client participation in all stages of the intervention can usefully involve "homework" assignments of various kinds, and/or exercises done during the sessions.
7. In working with groups, workers must balance leadership activity with facilitation work to ensure that all members participate according to their needs.
8. The action plan must make sense to all members of the client group, and must be seen by them as realistic.

9. In implementing the action plan, the allocation of tasks must take into account all aspects of what may be considered "capacities" in the broadest sense.
10. The first tasks of the action plan need to be ones that have a good possibility of being successful. This builds confidence for undertaking more challenging tasks later.

REFERENCES

Augsburger, David. This quote is invaluable to me, but I have been unable to trace its date or origin.

Corey, Marianne Schneider and Gerald Corey. (1993). *Becoming a Helper, Second Edition*. Pacific Grove, CA: Brooks/Cole Publishing Company.

Germain, Carel B. and Alex Gitterman. (1980). *The Life Model of Social Work Practice*. New York: Columbia University Press.

Middleton-Moz, Jane. (1994). Personal communication at a workshop presented in Sudbury, ON, Canada.

Siporin, Max. (1975). *Introduction to Social Work Practice*. New York: Macmillan Publishing Co., Inc.

Chapter 13

Empowerment:
Helping People Take Control
of Their Lives

Over the last twenty-five years social work literature has increasingly emphasized empowerment as a professional value and a method principle. The profession has effectively incorporated it into individual, group, and community practice (Simon, 1990:31). It is closely related to–but it is more than simply an application of–the principles of client self-determination and of involving the client actively in the helping process.

The adoption of these three principles has marked an important aspect of the profession's move away from the paternalistic influence of the so-called "medical model," which clinical practice adopted in the 1940s and 1950s. This model was attractive to the profession at least in part because, compared to the many successes of progressive medical treatments, social work appeared to lack the ability to "cure" or to "prevent" the psychosocial ills we set out to "correct." Borrowing from the medical profession led us to a style of practice, particularly in clinical settings, that set the worker up as the "expert" vis-à-vis the client. This led to a mode of intervention with individuals in which, albeit with good intentions, we tended to make the client the recipient of our solutions to their difficulties, rather than eliciting their active participation in the work of effecting change.

Our movement to a different professional focus stemmed in part from our realization of what Tyler, Pargament, and Gatz describe as

> a basic incongruity between the roles of helping relationships which involve [the professionals] as expert and their clients as dependent, and the goal of those relationships which is to foster the clients' independence. (1983:388)

Second, the profession as a whole was faced with the turmoil of the 1960s, including significant national reports on poverty, civil riots in protest against war and racism, the rebellion of the young against traditional values, and so on. The incorporation of systems theory into our professional thinking gave us a structured and meaningful framework for understanding many of the difficulties our clients brought to us. We returned to our earlier roots in looking at the interaction between people and their immediate and wider environments as influential in their struggles; we also returned to looking at what was systemic and structural–socially, politically, and economically–in the difficulties they were facing. In the words of some, we began to "put the 'social' back into social work."

Since so many of our clients came from the disadvantaged and marginalized groups of society, it became clear that a major part of the difficulty for many was a feeling of powerlessness: the conviction that no action of theirs could improve their lives. Furthermore, we started to examine whether we as professionals were in fact contributing to this feeling of powerlessness.

Third, the recognition of a common base of value, purpose, and method in all three areas of practice (Bartlett, 1970) led us back to a generic teaching model. In my opinion, this also played at least an indirect role in the practice implementation of the new professional focus. We saw, for instance, how individual change could be constructively fostered and enhanced by peer group support. From this threefold base we began to look creatively at the meaning of powerlessness to our clients and of how it could be overcome.

Pinderhughes (1983), contemplating the concept of power, quotes Basch, who says that:

> Throughout life the feeling of controlling one's destiny to some reasonable extent is the essential, psychological component of all aspects of life. (Basch, in Anthony and Benedek, 1975:513)

Looking at the socioeconomic and sociopolitical backgrounds of most of our clients, it is clear that this "essential component" is missing from their lives.

Staples states that "powerlessness is structural and social in origin and nature" (1990:32). From a similar base Solomon (1976) has identified three potential sources of powerlessness:

- negative self-evaluation attitudes of oppressed people toward themselves;
- negative experiences in the interaction between the victims of oppression and the outside systems which impinge upon them; and
- larger environmental systems which consistently block and deny effective action taking by powerless groups. (cited in Parsons, 1991:11)

The first is strongly reenforced by the North American conviction that poverty and disadvantage are the result of individual inadequacy. The second highlights the many defeats the poor and disadvantaged suffer at the hands of their immediate environment when they seek to change their life situation. Examples include a lack of marketable skills (which leads to repeated rejection in attempts to improve their employment status) and lack of information about where to get unbiased information about civil and legal rights in day-to-day life.

The third source of powerlessness sums up what experience from the 1960s to the present has demonstrated as a "given": the virtual impossibility for disadvantaged people to reach the power centers in society, and the impossibility of being heard by the decision makers at any government level. In the last twenty years there has been a political swing toward restrictions on the allocation of funds and services for the poor, making their lives even more harsh and hopeless. If we are to help them in their life situations, we must be more thoughtful in this regard in our professional encounters, and incorporate some level of empowerment into our practice thinking and method.

Hasenfeld states that:

A theory of empowerment is based on the assumption that the capacity of people to improve their lives is determined by their ability to control their environment, namely by having power. (1987:478)

The same author reminds us that in the social work encounter

> the difference in resources that worker and client bring to the
> issue to be resolved, of itself constitutes an undermining of
> empowerment for the client. (1987:470)

Our power of expertise, our power in interpersonal skills, and–to
a limited degree–our power of control over what the agency can and
will provide, apply to all our clients, whatever their socioeconomic
status, age, gender, or ethnic background (Hasenfeld, 1987:471).
Unless we are careful in our professional role we can actually contribute to the clients' sense of powerlessness by the manner in which
we provide service. Pinderhughes warns that even our compassion,
if we are not careful, can lead us into "pity" and a kind of practice
that perpetuates the institutional concept of social work as "philanthropy" offered by the successful to the victims of an indifferent
society (1983:337). This will require vigilant self-awareness, and,
as will be described below, some rethinking of our professional
focus and method (Gutierrez, 1990:152).

Hasenfeld highlights several areas in which a basic inequality of
power is a built-in aspect of most social work services. He speaks of
clients' lack of choice of which agency will best meet their needs
(1987:473-474). Some clients, of course, are assigned to specific
agencies by legal requirements–for example, social assistance, child
welfare, probation, and parole. But even voluntary clients are
restricted to some degree in their choice of agency by the various
agencies' separate categories of service.

In every case, the agency's mandate and administration determine
what resources are made available to the client (Hasenfeld, 1987:
474-475). Even when seeking service voluntarily, clients rarely
have any choice about the worker to whom they are initially
assigned. Some family service agencies are able to discuss the clients' preference for a male or female worker for marriage counseling; or an age and/or gender preference may be taken into account
for troubled adolescents, or for women recovering from sexual
assault or childhood sexual abuse perpetrated by a male. But most
agencies, and particularly the public ones, base the decision about
assigning workers on administrative factors such as caseload size,

agency-identified special skills of workers, geographic location of the client's residence, and so on.

We need to examine and become fully aware of how this administrative framework disempowers those who need and/or are eligible for social work services. Without such examination we may be perpetuating our own part in the systemic oppression of those whom we are committed to serve.

AN EMPOWERMENT FOCUS

Dodd and Gutierrez suggest that

> Social workers must give up their expert power and recognize that clients are the experts in regard to their own problems, capacities and potential solutions. (1990:69)

Breton suggests that this requires our intervention to be "collaborative participation"; a style of practice

> in which professional and the disempowered are differentially but equally involved as partners all along the process [of change.] (Breton, 1994:30)

These concepts are well illustrated in a study of welfare administration in Virginia Beach. The agency reviewed the manner in which financial aid to the needy was administered, and involved input from both clients and workers. Mumma's report of this project is illuminating, in that it was clear that neither workers nor clients felt good about the intake interview; speed and accuracy were emphasized at the expense of job satisfaction for the workers, and it was humiliating for the clients (1989:15).

Clients reported that

> they felt they were "failures" and did not give themselves credit for many skills and strengths they had developed and used while on financial aid. . . . For some the need for financial assistance was disabling . . . [and] had further eroded their self-confidence and sense of personal control. (1989:16)

As a result of this study, the eligibility interview was revised with the objective of providing a more hopeful approach and to help clients "view financial aid as a part of their own plans for self-sufficiency" (1989:20).

Five objectives were identified as being significant in an empowering approach to this group of clients: honest and genuine validation of the person; skill identification to counteract "failure" self-perception; future orientation (moving toward goal achievement); redirecting or confirming the client's perspective; and initiating manageable steps toward greater objectives and goals (1989:19-20).

These objectives form the basis of empowerment practice. It would be foolish to argue that empowerment practice has been made easier, especially since the prevailing North American trend has been to reduce or withdraw government support of many social services to the most needful citizens. But for that very reason it is important to practice empowerment to the highest degree possible— and there is always some degree of possibility.

Practice Applications

Hasenfeld states categorically that

> . . . the major function of social work [is] empowering people to be able to make choices and gain control over their environment. (1987:478)

Once we recognize the power difference in our professional contacts, we need to approach each client or group with awareness of its meaning for them. Dodd and Gutierrez elaborate on Breton's statement (above), stating that

> The worker must perceive him/herself as enabler, organizer, consultant, compatriot with the client, [so as not to replicate] the powerlessness which clients experience with other helpers and professionals. (1990:69)

These statements provide us with a position from which we can begin to empower our clients. From the first moment of contact we need to speak and behave in ways that provide a climate in which clients feel that we do not see them as helpless; that we respect what they bring to the helping process; and that our aim is to help them find what they believe they need to take control of their lives. We create this climate through our "genuineness, [giving a sense of] mutual respect, open communication and informality" (Gutierrez, 1990:151). This will help to lessen the clients' sense of inequality of power noted above, and will promote their confidence in expressing their view of the issues and possible solutions.

Gutierrez (1990:149) and Rappaport, (1985:21) identify five techniques for empowering clients:

(i) accepting the clients' definition of the problem;
(ii) identifying and building upon existing strengths;
(iii) engaging in a power analysis of the client's situation;

Citing this last as critical, Gutierrez elaborates the process:

a. How are conditions of powerlessness affecting the client's situation?
b. Identify sources of potential power in the client's situation.
c. Dialogue aimed at exploring and identifying the social structure origins of the client's current situation.

(iv) teaching specific skills; and
(v) mobilizing resources and advocating for the client. (1990: 152)

We need to be creative in our thinking about the application of empowerment in all areas of practice. Two examples from clinical practice follow.

Mrs. Eleanor Jackson, aged seventy-six, was referred by her family physician to the social services of the local housing administration in a small city (population 90,000). She had moved into Ridgeview Gardens, a new apartment block for seniors recently set up by the city's housing committee. There were fifty apartments on four floors.

Dr. Ziegler stated that Mrs. Jackson was mildly depressed and having anxiety attacks. This was affecting her sleep patterns and made it very difficult for her to go outdoors alone, even to buy groceries.

She recently gave up her home in a small town about 200 miles away, where she had lived for over fifty years. She had managed well alone since her husband died fourteen years ago, but the housework and yard work had become too much for her.

One son lives here in the city. He and his wife both work full-time outside the home and they have three young children. Dr. Ziegler feels they have made it clear to Mrs. Jackson that she cannot depend on them too much. A daughter is married and lives on the West Coast, but she has virtually cut herself off from her mother and the family since the father's death.

Dr. Ziegler prescribed a limited amount of a mild sleeping pill, but was reluctant to prescribe antidepressant medication at this time. She found Mrs. Jackson to be in good physical health and felt that what she needed was "someone to talk to about her fears."

At the first meeting with Mrs. Jackson, Marguerite, an experienced worker with the housing administration, found her to be a well-groomed older woman, physically agile and mentally alert. She spoke with very flat affect. Her apartment was neat and obviously well-kept; the furnishings were in good condition.

The worker learned that Mrs. Jackson's son had suggested that she move to the city to "be near them if anything happened." Her next-door neighbors of many years, along with their daughter and son-in-law, had helped her organize the sale of some of her things, and in arranging the move. Her son had paid for a young woman here to come in for several days to help her unpack and get settled. In describing this, in spite of a very flat emotional tone, Mrs. Jackson came across as having taken an active part in all these activities.

Mrs. Jackson said that she had not had a good night's sleep since she moved here. She was awakened by every sound and got up to check the front and patio doors several times during the night. (Her apartment was on the second floor.) When she had to go out she was very anxious much of the time. Taking the bus and shopping in the supermarket sometimes made her so frightened that she had to check out and leave before she had completed her list. Once, while doing her banking, she was so overwhelmed that she had to ask the staff to call a taxi to take her home.

She had not made more than a passing acquaintance of any of her neighbors in the apartments. She believed they "all grew up and have lived here all their lives, so they know each other well." She does not want to "intrude" on them and besides, she "does not know what kind of people they are."

The worker asked what Mrs. Jackson thought would help her–what would make a difference. She said that Dr. Ziegler just did not seem to understand that she is too ill to live independently any more. She did not realize it herself until she moved here, but she felt now that she needed nursing home care. She had never had a woman doctor before, and although Dr. Ziegler "speaks nicely" and had been in touch with her previous doctor, Mrs. Jackson felt she "doesn't understand my case."

In empowerment terms the worker could accept Mrs. Jackson's definition of the problem. She was clearly saying she needed more care and attention and this was not available in her new apartment. In recognizing her stated wish to enter a nursing home, Marguerite was careful not to overemphasize the doctor's assessment of her general good health, lest this came across as minimizing how debilitated she really feels.

Taking her expressed need for more care and attention as a starting point, the worker recognized with Mrs. Jackson how very difficult it has been for her to make this move–leaving friends of many years, familiar stores, bus routes, having to change doctors, and so on. Mrs. Jackson began to cry and said that indeed it had been hard. She even had to part with her beloved old cat–pets were not allowed in this building. She missed her bridge group and said bridge had always been an important pastime.

The day before this visit, Marguerite had received a call from the daughter of another resident who was concerned for her mother's well-being while she–the daughter–would be away for two weeks. Her mother, Mrs. Gooderham, had been back in her apartment for four weeks, after having hip replacement surgery and rehabilitation care. She was making a good recovery but her daughter had made a habit of calling her every morning and evening to check that everything was okay. Her daughter felt she had come to rely on the daily phone calls for reassurance.

Marguerite had had plans that once the Gardens was fully occupied she would suggest a meeting at which the residents could talk about forming a council. Although the building was not yet full, she decided to schedule a first meeting that week. She offered to take Mrs. Jackson to the meeting, which was going to be held in the basement recreation room of the building. In discussing the council plan, Marguerite emphasized that most of the residents did not know each other before they moved in; they came from many different areas of this large city, and some, like herself, from other centers. This meeting would introduce her to some of the other residents, and she assured Mrs. J that if she became anxious she could always leave.

At the meeting (with Mrs. Gooderham's permission), the worker raised the question of a twice daily call to make sure that she was managing okay, for the sake of her daughter's peace of mind. Several residents volunteered for this. One woman said she had heard of a seniors' apartment building where they have a "buddy" system. Each floor is organized so that "buddies" take turns calling each other, morning and evening, every day. If you do not get your call, you go and check your buddy; likewise if he or she does not answer your call, you check on your buddy, getting help if necessary from the superintendent. The woman who suggested this said half-humorously that as they are all "not getting any younger" it would not hurt to set this up at the Gardens. Mr. Demille said it might be a relief to his daughter. "She's always bugging me to go live with her so that she wouldn't worry so much," he said. He valued his independence and was not ready to give it up yet. The worker fully supported their implementing this plan.

In reply to a request for other ideas that might make life easier for them, another resident suggested that for those who did not drive, especially in the winter months, a registry could be set up for people to share taxis to go for groceries. Another resident, a car-owner, spoke up and talked about a car pool for grocery shopping. They could have a "registry" and a weekly fee to share the cost of gas. This would help them all. Mrs. Kohl had heard that a supermarket in Jarvistown, where her brother lived, had agreed to run a weekly bus picking up seniors from nearby residences for grocery shopping. Three members offered to get together and look into this possibility with the local supermarket, but the car pool idea really took hold, and two residents had started a register of car owners before the meeting ended.

Mrs. Jackson stayed for the whole meeting, and when asked, she helped with the dishes afterwards. The worker noticed that she was very shy and quiet most of the time, with many anxious hand gestures. Mrs. Carlucci, a very outgoing woman sitting next to her, tried to draw her out, but Marguerite could see how easy it would be for the residents to mistake Mrs. Jacksons's shyness for standoffishness and thus leave her alone.

At first Mrs. Jackson said she did not think the "buddy" system applied to her, but apparently a few days later Mrs. Zymanski from down the hall asked her to be a "buddy" for her, and so she joined in. Two weeks later she told Marguerite that this buddy system with Mrs. Z and the car pool arrangement for grocery shopping had made a difference. She was still nervous at night, but during the day she felt a little better. She said she was still very lonely, however, and missed her friends.

Following the schema outlined by Gutierrez and Rappaport, Marguerite focused on what steps Mrs. Jackson might take to overcome her feeling that she was very much alone, and that nobody really cared about her. Could she perhaps ask around—put up a sign in the laundromat, for instance—about bridge players in the building? She was reluctant.—"It is difficult to start playing with people you don't know," she said. The worker reminded her that she knows she is a good player, and others would appreciate this. Eventually Mrs. Jackson spoke about this to Mrs. Zymanski, who knew of three keen players who had been looking for a fourth.

After a while she confided to Mrs. Zymanski about her nervousness at night. She learned that Mrs. Zymanski had had her phone moved from the kitchen to beside her bed, and it had given her a sense of security at night. Mrs. Zymanski helped Mrs. Jackson arrange this and it made quite a difference for her.

As time went on, the residents began to develop a sense of community. Some showed effective leadership skills and the Residents' Council became an important factor in their feeling of having a voice in administrative matters. Marguerite suggested that from then on she would only attend when they felt she could be helpful in some way, and all agreed to this.

Mrs. Jackson learned that many of the residents, like herself, had not known each other before they moved in. She realized that she could take some initiative in inviting them to her apartment for morning coffee, taking her turn to have bridge club at her place, and so on. Not long after this, Mrs. Jackson helped Mrs. Carlucci and Mr. Garfield organize a cards and games afternoon that was well attended and was planned to become a regular event.

At a recent Residents' Council meeting three residents who had known each other before they moved in and knew the city well, said they had not realized how strange it must have been for others not so fortunate, and they began to discuss the formation of a "Welcoming Committee" (Scharlach, 1985: 35-46). They asked Mrs. Jackson and others for their ideas and as a result were considering providing newcomers with a kit to include a city map, a list of bus routes, and suggestions about advantageous shopping, as well as planning more personal welcoming efforts within the Gardens community.

Discussion

Parsons states that the empowerment approach, if it is to be effective, focuses on developing the following five qualities in the person or group:

(i) the development of attitudes and beliefs about one's efficacy to take action;

(ii) the development of critical thinking about one's world;

(iii) the acquisition of knowledge and skills needed to take action;

(iv) support and mutual aid of one's peers in any given situation; and

(v) the taking of action to make change in the face of impinging problems. (1991:12)

Examining the outcome of the work with Mrs. Jackson, it is clear that the worker helped her

(i) To change her attitude about what she could do in the situation; i.e., join in the Residents' Council, the buddy system, and the shopping car pool; move her phone; utilize her skill at bridge to engage neighbors in an activity she enjoyed, thereby giving her a reason to invite them to her apartment.

(ii) To reexamine her assumption that she was the only resident who did not know anyone before moving in; that some of her needs for friendly support could be met without resorting to a nursing home; and furthermore, that there were congenial people at the Gardens.

(iii) To acquire knowledge and skills needed to take action, by observing and hearing the suggestions of others about the buddy system, the car pool for shopping, and the Welcoming Committee.

(iv) Linking her into the Residents' Council helped her to realize that she was not alone with her feelings but could receive others' support and practical help.

(v) This led her to eventually take part in various actions designed to solve her immediate difficulties. Successful outcomes there will lead to greater confidence when future problems arise.

Some aspects of Mrs. Jackson's difficulty illustrate the importance of what Germain and Gitterman call the "goodness-of-fit" concept. This refers to the balance between the needs of the system and the available environmental resources (1980: 80). Pinderhughes states that "when the environment in which people live is nutritive, they flourish," and elaborates this, saying that

> Healthy environments provide the necessary resources of protection, security, support and supplies at the appropriate time and in the appropriate way. (1983:332)

Mrs. Jackson had managed well and adapted to widowhood in the familiar physical and social surroundings of the small town where she had lived for so many years. Uprooted and placed in a setting that had none of the supportive aspects of her hometown, "forced to rely on her own inner resources" (Pinderhughes, 1983:333) and finding them inadequate, she became virtually unable to function and felt completely helpless. Had her son and daughter-in-law been more considerate of what this change meant for her, and had they initially been more emotionally and practically supportive, Mrs. Jackson may have been able to adapt more readily. It is interesting that she was able to function appropriately in one area: her house-keeping; the only setting in which she was surrounded by familiar objects and where she felt in control.

It is probably partly a reflection of her age, and of having to relocate on her own for the first time in fifty years, that she could not find the necessary inner resources to cope effectively with her new situation. The solution this hitherto competent elder woman sought—entry into a nursing home—was a result of her belief that she could not function and needed to surrender to others the whole burden of responsibility for choices, decisions, and actions in the unfamiliar surroundings.

One further point is significant. The worker's empowerment thinking and a solution focus, in linking this woman to immediately accessible environmental resources, helped her to become a full participant in taking action to meet some of her felt needs. The approach taken here recognized, but did not emphasize, Mrs. Jackson's struggle to deal with her immediate losses, nor did it explore the roots of some apparent estrangement from her children, particularly her daughter. While these probably played a part in her depression, the worker's focus helped to repair her damaged self-esteem, and gave her a greater feeling of control over her situation. The worker also focused on creating some changes that created a more supportive environment.

Another clinical example is described by Haney (1988), in his personal story of learning to live with AIDS. Haney describes the feelings of total helplessness that flood the being of the person when first diagnosed with AIDS. He identifies the feelings of blame that others attach to the diagnosis, the sense that those who have AIDS are

> some fringe element "out there," an element unworthy of compassion because of some character flaw or inappropriate behavior. (1988:251)

He cites the sense that AIDS brings of being disconnected from important aspects of life:

> . . . our loved ones; from ways we have of defining ourselves, such as job activities, capabilities, skills and physical appearance. Finally . . . a disconnection from . . . a sense of power and control over our lives, hopes, dreams and aspirations. (1988:251)

Out of his own experience, Haney offers six ways of providing empowerment to persons with AIDS. First, he identifies the importance of helping the person focus on what positive consequences can come out of even such a negative experience. This can be done by presenting to the person evidence that some people with AIDS do live longer than their doctors have predicted. He quotes one person who confided to him that "I need help to focus on living with AIDS, not dying with dignity" (1988:252). Second, he emphasizes the vital importance of a support group. He says, "It was through attending my first support group that I found the beginning of hope" (1988:252), and stresses that if persons with AIDS have no support group, it is the social workers' duty to help them find caring people.

Third, the matter of reconnection is vital in recovering a sense of self-worth—perhaps through a part-time job where flexibility of hours could accommodate the person's variable levels of energy.

Next, Haney states that social workers can help the person with AIDS access information about different medical and nontraditional medical services to "provide persons with AIDS with ways to control their illness and their lives." This, he states, gives them "keys to not giving up." He adds that "a sense of power and control is an integral part of providing empowerment to persons with AIDS" (1988:252).

Lastly, Haney reminds us that advocacy is an important element in our help to this group of persons. "It is empowering, reassuring, and truly beneficial to know help is there when it's needed [to] advocate for our needs and our rights" (1988:253).

Haney's discussion and Mrs. Jackson's case emphasize the integral part that linkage with support groups plays in the empowerment process. Lee (1990), Breton (1988), and Simon (1990) also point this out.

EMPOWERMENT IN COMMUNITY PRACTICE

In her valuable discussion of empowerment-oriented practice, Breton states that "groups are natural vehicles for empowerment" (1994:30), particularly in work with oppressed groups whose empowerment has a social action component. Breton continues:

> The strength in numbers phenomenon, as an element of mutual aid, must be activated for the purpose of facilitating social action and attaining social justice. (1994:31)

Social workers can be involved in various undertakings with groups of people who want to take concerted action for the benefit of their community, but feel powerless to achieve their objectives.

> Tenants in a medium-size, low-rental housing project formed an Association initially to petition the local housing administration to repair and/or replace worn-out playground equipment. However, as the group got going, different concerns were raised. Some wanted to institute a weekly, voluntary clean-up system to keep the lanes and pathways clean and free of debris; others did not see this as a priority, but rather emphasized the need for improved lighting of the same lanes and pathways, where many female residents felt unsafe walking after dark. Another group wanted to press for a total indoor and outdoor paint and repair job throughout the project, which had become shabby and run-down over the years of its existence. This predominantly black, low-income group felt there was no real hope of their achieving any of these goals on their

own and appealed to the housing administration's social worker to help them. Chris was the social worker for this housing project.

Part of the social worker's obligation here was to help the group prioritize their concerns, and in so doing facilitate the kind of exchange of views that would alleviate conflict and power struggles. This was not easy. The association was divided strongly on the issues, and Chris helped them recognize that such conflicts would seriously weaken their position as they made application to the housing authority for any of the desired changes.

Chris recognized that these people felt there was some danger for them in "taking on the landlord" (Kuyek, 1995). This perception was a reality for them. He suggested that once they agreed on their priorities they had strength of numbers in their favor. (Breton, 1994:31)

Discussion

It would be important for this worker not to give them false reassurance that "environments can always be manipulated in [the petitioners'] favor" (1988:48). But both Breton (1988) and Kuyek (1990) urge us not to play into a defeatist attitude. Breton urges us "not to settle for less than doing whatever it is possible to do" (1988:48), and Kuyek says that "too often we limit our demands to what the power structures will allow us to have" (1990:149).

Following Kuyek's outline, the worker could suggest that the group members begin by asking themselves:

> What do you really want? What would the ideal situation look like? What would have to happen to achieve the ideal situation? What is in the way? Is there a reason why you should not ask for the ideal situation? What would happen if you did? (1990:148)

Kuyek's questions bring a component of practical reality that can make the undertaking feel more manageable. The long-standing technique of breaking the task down into what someone has called bite-sized pieces is as effective here as it is in clinical practice.

Returning to the case:

> In the course of several meetings, the Association came together, agreeing that the plan of organizing voluntary clean-up of the lanes and pathways could be offered as proof of their readiness to take some responsibility themselves and of their "not asking for the moon," as one member said. They further agreed that their priorities were the playground equipment and improved lighting, and that both were of equal importance. One member suggested that they could certainly recommend that the administration conduct a survey of the whole property, specifically the condition of exterior and interior paint and repairs. Some of the more timid members were anxious that this might indeed be "asking for the moon," and that their request would have unpleasant repercussions, but Mr. Johnson (a resident) said he believed it would depend on how it was presented, and several others agreed.
>
> As the plans progressed, Mr. Johnson and three others showed themselves to have good leadership skills, and Chris began to function simply as a resource person. The association sought his advice about the manner of their presentation, and precisely to whom it should be addressed, but agreed that they did not need him to be present when this was done.
>
> After receiving these requests, the Housing Maintenance Committee asked Chris for his opinion. He was able to support the tenants by describing the deplorable—even unsafe—condition of the playground equipment; since he had visited the project after dark, he was also able to describe the inadequate lighting. The Committee agreed to prepare cost estimates of these two improvements—which seemed likely to be within the yearly budget—and submit them to the city with their support of these requests' validity.
>
> The Administration dismissed the paint and repairs request as excessive. However, one of the members of the Housing Maintenance Committee later went over to look at the playground. He observed the condition of the exterior of the adjoining buildings and told Chris he was going to bring this up again—perhaps with modifications—once they had permis-

sion to work on the playground and lighting. He was not very hopeful, however, because of what he called the current "wrong-headed, 'cut back on everything' thinking."

Discussion

One of the important tasks of the community social worker is helping the group identify and develop indigenous leadership. True empowerment must lead here, as in clinical practice, to the system's being able to function effectively without our help. Time limitations add a healthy degree of urgency to the implementation of this objective, perhaps especially in community practice.

In their significant report on community empowerment strategies, Fawcett et al. list eight elements involved in "training new behaviors to increase the effectiveness of community group leaders and individual citizens" (1984:147). Specifically, these authors state that the ability to produce empowerment objectives may be a function of:

- knowledge of problems and solution alternatives;
- skill in presenting issues and implementing other empowerment tactics;
- capacity to control consequences for critical actors in the system, e.g., positive: votes for elected officials or negative: unfavorable newspaper reports; and
- structural variables, such as the opportunity to gain access to agendas of meetings of elected officials. (1984:146-147)

Thus, in further discussion of effective empowerment goals in the case examples they describe, these authors add that it is necessary, among other strategies, to:

- increase knowledge of community problems [among] those most affected by the problems;
- increase knowledge of the possible consequences of projects proposed by persons outside the affected community;
- train new behaviors in order to increase the effectiveness of community group leaders and individual citizens; and

- obtain and communicate information to influence public policies regarding the distribution of resources. (adapted from
  Fawcett et al., 1984:147-149)

These authors describe seven community projects, some concerning social action on a wider scale than the case example cited above.
They designed "social technologies," i.e., replicable procedural
tools having the objective of enhancing "control by community
members over important aspects of their lives" (1984:148).

In their example of "Increasing Knowledge About the Possible
Impacts of Proposed Roadway Projects on Neighborhoods," these
authors developed a "Consequence Analysis method" to obtain
input from representative neighborhood residents indicating what
they saw as the possible consequences for them of a roadway-build-
ing project in their neighborhood. When this guide was circulated to
a majority of residents, it was found that the rate of their opposition
to the project increased measurably as a result of the new information (1984:153-154).

The responses were compiled and forwarded to the decision makers in charge of the building project. These authors report that this
Consequence Analysis method

> was judged to be a small, but significant contribution to the
> neighborhood association's ultimately successful efforts to halt
> construction of the roadway. (1984:154)

Social workers do not always have the kind of independent
agency sponsorship (a university-sponsored research project, for
example) and the resources that were available to Fawcett and his
colleagues. Nevertheless, we can take their seven constituents, listed
above, as a sound basis for effective empowerment of community
groups in various projects. In many instances, we may have to
employ less sophisticated methods, and we must be prepared for a
less formal process of informing the community. But we may be
able to help them organize for action, by seeking out the support of
powerful persons–locally elected representatives, perhaps–who may
be persuaded to speak for them in the decision-making arena.

The key to a practice imbued with empowerment thinking and
methods will lie first in self-awareness about our perception of our

professional role. We need to examine carefully our attitude toward those clients who present with feelings of "failure," of hopelessness and helplessness; we need to look at our own need to be the "rescuer" or the "expert"; and we need to avoid the trap of "pity and philanthropy" cited by Pinderhughes (1983:152). Second, we must be creative in finding ways to share the tasks of effecting change with our clients, individuals, families, groups, and communities, such that they regain a sense of having control over their lives. This sense of control is the element that several writers cited here have identified as essential in personal well-being.

SUMMARY OF MAIN POINTS

1. The principle of empowerment requires that we stop thinking of the professional relationship as being one of worker as "expert" and client as "recipient." Client(s) are the experts on their life situation.
2. We must be alert to prevent, as far as possible, the traditional structures of service provision from replicating the pattern of power deprivation that so many of our clients feel in other significant areas of their lives.
3. Restoring self-esteem is integral to empowerment practice. The North American emphasis on individual success as being solely a matter of adequate effort and industry contributes forcefully to the low self-esteem of those who do not "make it" in our society.
4. We need to be genuine in conveying respect for clients, and we need to identify with them the skills they clearly demonstrate but perhaps undervalue.
5. There are structural and systemic obstacles—social, economic, and political—in the path of many of those who seek our services to improve their life situation. We need to recognize these and work with our clients to surmount them.
6. Many of our clients are virtually excluded from access to the decision-making levels of our society. Part of our role needs to be as a source of information and advocacy to change this.

7. Our advocacy can be an important source of strength to individuals and groups who are struggling with feelings of powerlessness.

8. Empowerment thinking and methods can be valuable in clinical practice and with multiclient systems.

9. Support groups are a vital factor in empowerment in all areas of practice.

10. What one writer has called "collaborative strategies" are significant methods in empowerment practice, i.e., an emphasis on sharing the tasks of effecting change.

REFERENCES

Bartlett, Harriett M. (1970). *The Common Base of Social Work Practice.* Washington, DC: National Association of Social Workers.

Basch, Michael. (1975). In *Depression and Human Existence.* (1975). E. James Anthony and Theresa Benedek, eds. Boston: Little, Brown and Co., p. 513. Cited in Pinderhughes, 1983:331.

Breton, Margot. (1988). "The Need for Mutual Aid Groups in a Drop-in for Homeless Women: The Sistering Case." *Social Work with Groups*, 11(4): 47-61.

————. (1994). "On the Meaning of Empowerment and Empowerment-Oriented Social Work Practice." *Social Work with Groups*, 17(3):23-37.

Dodd, Pamela and Lorraine Gutierrez. (1990). "Preparing Students for the Future: A power perspective on community practice." *Administration in Social Work*, 14(2):63-78.

Fawcett, Stephen B., Tom Seekins, Paula L. Whang, Charles Muiu, and Yolanda Suarez de Balcazar. (1984). "Creating and Using Technologies for Community Empowerment." In *Studies in Empowerment: Steps Toward Understanding and Action.* Julian Rappaport and R. Hess, eds. Binghamton, New York: The Haworth Press.

Germain, Carel B. and Alex Gitterman. (1980). *The Life Model of Social Work Practice.* New York: Columbia University Press.

Gutierrez, Lorraine. (1990). "Working with Women of Color: An Empowerment Perspective." *Social Work*, 35(2):149-153.

Haney, Patrick. (1988). "Providing Empowerment to the Person with AIDS." *Social Work*, 33(3):251-253.

Hasenfeld, Yeheskel. (1987). "Power in Social Work Practice." *Social Service Review*, 61:469-483.

Kuyek, Joan Newman. (1990). *Fighting for Hope: Organizing to Realize our Dreams.* Montreal: Black Rose Books.

————. (1995). Personal communication.

Lee, Judith A.B. (1990). "Return to our Roots." *Social Work with Groups*, 11(4): 5-9.

Mumma, Edward. (1989). "Reform at the Local Level: Virginia Beach Empowers Both Clients and Workers." *Public Welfare*, 47(2):15-24.

Parsons, Ruth J. (1991). "Empowerment: Purpose and Practice Principle in Social Work." *Social Work with Groups*, 14(2):7-21.

Pinderhughes, Elaine B. (1983). "Empowerment for our Clients and for Ourselves." *Social Casework*, 64(6):331-338.

Rappaport, Julian (1985). "The Power of Empowerment Language." *Social Policy*, 16(2):15-21.

Scharlach, Andrew E. (1985). "Social Group-Work with Institutionalized Elders: A Task-Centered Approach." *Social Work with Groups*, 8(3):33-47.

Simon, Barbara Levy. (1990). "Rethinking Empowerment." *Journal of Progressive Human Services*, 1(1):27-39.

Solomon, Barbara. (1976). *Black Empowerment: Social Work in Oppressed Communities*. New York: Columbia University Press. Cited in Parsons, 1991:11.

Staples, Lee H. (1990). "Powerful Ideas about Empowerment." *Administration in Social Work*, 14(2):29-42.

Tyler, Forrest B., Kenneth I. Pargament, and Margaret Gatz. (1983). "The Resource Collaborator Role: A Mode for Interactions Involving Psychologists." *American Psychologist*, 38(4):388-398.

OTHER USEFUL READING

Kieffer, Charles H. (1984). "Citizen Empowerment: A Developmental Perspective." In *Studies in Empowerment: Steps Toward Understanding and Action*. Binghamton, New York: The Haworth Press.

Longres, John F. and Eileen McLeod. (1980). "Consciousness Raising and Social Work Practice." *Social Casework*, 61(5):267-276.

Index

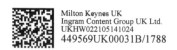

9 780789 001887